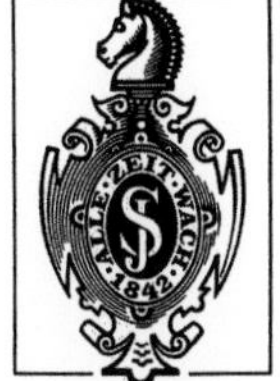

Roland R. Schmoker

Functional Reconstruction of the Mandible

Experimental Foundations and
Clinical Experience

With a Foreword by M. E. Müller

With 79 Figures

Springer-Verlag Berlin Heidelberg New York
London Paris Tokyo

Dr. Dr. ROLAND R. SCHMOKER
Spezialarzt FMH für Plastische
und Wiederherstellungs-Chirurgie
Lindenhofspital
CH-3012 Bern

Translator:

TERRY C. TELGER
6112 Waco Way
Ft. Worth, TX 76133, USA

This book resulted from the collaboration of the Department of Maxillofacial Surgery of the University of Basel and the Department of Reconstructive and Plastic Surgery, the Department of Experimental Surgery, the Domestic Animal and Horse Clinic, and the Bone Histology Laboratory of the Anatomical Institute of the University of Bern. The work was supported by the Research Promotion Fund of the Working Committee for Osteosynthesis and by the Schweizerischer Nationalfonds.

Title of the German Edition
R. Schmoker: Die funktionelle Unterkieferrekonstruktion
© Springer-Verlag Berlin Heidelberg 1986

ISBN-13: 978-3-642-71758-1   e-ISBN-13: 978-3-642-71756-7
DOI: 10.1007/978-3-642-71756-7

Library of Congress Cataloging-in-Publication Data. Schmoker, R. (Roland), 1943–   . Functional reconstruction of the mandible. Translation of: Die Funktionelle Unterkieferrekonstruktion. Bibliography: p. Includes index. 1. Mandible—Surgery. 2. Mandibular prosthesis. 3. Surgery, Experimental. I. Title. [DNLM: 1. Mandible—Surgery. 2. Mandibular Prosthesis. WU 600 S356f] RD526.S3613 1987   617'.522   86-31529

2124/3130-543210

Foreword

Since 1958 the Association for the Study of Internal Fixation (ASIF) has worked to establish the experimental and biomechanical principles of the operative treatment of fractures. It has been proven that immediate, pain-free mobilization, made possible by stable internal fixation, is the key to restoring function in a fractured extremity. The same principles were applied in 1972/73 by Roland Schmoker, who developed a universal plate and sophisticated instrument set designed initially for the treatment of comminuted fractures of the mandible.

To extend the applications of his plate to reconstructions after extensive tumor resections, he supplemented the device with temporomandibular joint prostheses and anchoring elements for the attachment of dentures. He first tested the functional stability of these implants experimentally in sheep. Later he found that the minipig had a more human-like jaw shape and masticatory action, and so he tested the implants in 37 minipigs that underwent extensive mandibular resections without bone grafting, using sequential dye injections and postoperative weight gain to chart the progress of osseous regeneration. Seven other animals were not operated and served as controls.

These animal studies enabled Dr. Schmoker to make continual improvements in the implants and instrument set and also to refine the indications for intra- and extraoral procedures. All this laid the necessary groundwork for applying the method clinically after tumor resections. Because the anchoring elements that were tested in animals have not yet been employed in humans, the book must withhold a definitive assessment of their clinical potential.

The present monograph, which was supported by the promotional fund of the ASIF and by federal funds, makes an important contribution to the problem of restoring mandibular continuity after comminuted fractures and tumor resections. The work of Dr. Schmoker is significant from a research standpoint and contains many new ideas. It documents the scientific, experimental foundations of the now widely practiced procedure of stable internal fixation of the mandible. It also gives the oral and maxillofacial surgeon valuable practical guidelines for his operative procedures and offers new directions for further research.

Both the author and publisher are to be congratulated for this superbly illustrated and well presented work.

Bern   MAURICE E. MÜLLER

Table of Contents

Introduction

Osseous defects of the mandible can occur as a result of trauma (especially gunshot injuries), tumor resections, inflammatory diseases, and radionecrosis. A defect which disrupts the continuity of the bony mandibular arch or causes loss of the temporomandibular joint can cause difficulties with eating, speaking, respiration, and the containment of saliva, quite apart from the cosmetic deformity that is produced. These sequelae may occur primarily or they may be secondary to deviation of the mandibular stumps during cicatricial healing, in which case scar contraction can restrict the oral cavity and lead to prolapse of the tongue.

The causal treatment of these sequelae is based on the reestablishment of mandibular function by:

1. restoring the bony continuity of the mandible,
2. replacing the temporomandibular joint,
3. anchoring the dental prosthesis.

Functional stability depends on *restoring the continuity of the mandible* with regard to shape, stiffness, and load-bearing capacity. In very general terms we define this restoration as any motion-stable and preferably load-stable union of a fracture or defect that avoids the secondary effects of a temporary restriction of function (decreased joint motion, ankylosis, dystrophy, osteoporosis). Just as in surgery of the extremities, the concept of early mobilization has assumed major importance in reconstructive surgery of the mandible. However, we feel that most publications that deal with ways of stabilizing the mandibular stumps and techniques of bony anchorage violate the principles of functionally stable fixation that have evolved in surgery of the extremities. In many cases, for example, the fixation necessitates lengthy immobilization of the mandible by intermaxillary fixation (splinting the mandible to the maxilla). This immobilization compromises virtually all mandibular functions. The absence of a functional stimulus, moreover, can lead to the resorption of a bone graft that has been inserted to bridge an osseous defect. Without a viable bone graft, even modern internal fixation plates are unable to bridge a defect with adequate stability. This is due to the small dimensions of the plate, which are dictated by the requirements of malleability and the avoidance of stress protection, impingement on the overlying mucosa, and disruption of facial contour.

The design of internal fixation plates is based on the principle of fracture stabilization by compression, which requires that most of the stresses acting on the stabilized fracture be transferred across the fracture site as interfragmental pressure. If the bony buttress necessary for this transfer is lacking, the implant bridging the defect will have to transmit all the imposed stresses by itself. Bone plates are not stable enough to perform this function. We see this from the implant loosening that occurs with the resumption of masticatory function and from the malalignment of the mandibular stumps that occurs with scar contraction.

Concerning *replacement of the temporomandibular joint,* loss of this joint is uncommon, but if it does occur, the defect will lead to cicatricial or bony ankylosis. Surgical replacement of this joint is difficult because of the close proximity of large blood vessels, the root of the zygoma, and the facial nerve plexus. Also, it is difficult to achieve stable anchorage of a prosthesis in the thin articular process. We feel that many of the problems that remain unsolved today can be attributed largely to unfavorable conventional implant designs.

Denture fixation is a problem whenever an extensive mandibular defect exists. It is particularly difficult to reestablish masticatory function in the edentulous mandible, where an absence of retention makes it impossible to stabilize the denture adequately. When residual teeth are present, they may become loosened due to excessive loading.

A method for the temporary or permanent fixation of mandibular stumps in the presence of a mandibular defect must fulfill several requirements: stability under functional loading, retention of the mandibular stumps in an anatomically correct position, and the option of primary or secondary bone grafting. Moreover, devices which stabilize the mandible should be adjustable in all directions so that they will have universal adaptability. The dimensions of the implant must be small enough to permit the necessary revascularization of transplanted bone while avoiding impingement on the overlying skin and mucosa. Close spacing of the anchoring elements guarantees optimum fixation in a minimum of space.

In an effort to satisfy these requirements, we began in 1973 to develop our own appliances for mandibular reconstruction. We followed the principles of the ASIF (Association for the Study of Internal Fixation), working closely with the designer, Dr. R. MATHYS, and with the help of Prof. Dr. B. SPIESSL and Prof. Dr. H. TSCHOPP.

We were able to develop a reconstruction plate that was adjustable in three dimensions ("three-dimensionally bendable reconstruction plate," 3-DBRP), a condylar prosthesis, a reconstruction plate with condylar head, and anchoring elements for abutment posts. Practical use of the implants was tested in animal experiments. Our experience in this area will be presented and discussed on the basis of selected cases. A series of 21 consecutive patients operated over a 4-year period at the Department of Plastic and Reconstructive Surgery (Head: Prof. Dr. H. TSCHOPP) and the Visceral Surgical Clinic of the University of Bern (Head: Prof. Dr. R. BERCHTOLD) shows that while functional mandibular reconstruction is an infrequent procedure, it offers major benefits in terms of decreased morbidity and avoidance of debilitation owing to preservation of the temporomandibular joint and mandibular arch.

1 Historical Review

The earliest reports on partial mandibular resections were published in 1821 by
VON GRAEFE [43] and in 1823 by DEADERICK [32]. In 1929 BERGENFELDT [8] described the serious sequelae of more extensive mandibular resections, especially those involving the anterior portion of the arch. Loss of the anterior suspension of the tongue allows it to fall back and cause airway obstruction.
Another problem is muscular traction, which causes the stumps to deviate
medially and posteriorly and also to rotate on the frontal plane, producing a
lingual angulation of the teeth. Scar contraction causes further loss of space in
the oral cavity, leading ultimately to a forward prolapse of the tongue. Wire
ligatures, Kirschner wires, mesh trays, and plates − with or without bone grafting − all found clinical use as methods of stabilizing the mandibular stumps.

Kirschner wires and rods [5, 55, 62, 63, 65, 66, 124, 136] were used to secure
bone grafts (Fig. 1), to stabilize the mandibular stumps, and to support the soft
tissues. Stabilization after hemimandibulectomy was effected by seating the
implant into the glenoid fossa (Figs. 2−4), and after partial mandibular resection by interposing the implant between the bone ends (Figs. 5−8).

External fixation with transcutaneous pins was used both in its simplest
form (Fig. 9) and in more complex configurations, especially in the treatment
of fractures. It was less frequently used to stabilize mandibular stumps or bone
grafts in patients with mandibular defects [18, 37, 41, 49, 61, 83].

Precursors of the *metallic mesh trays* [40, 52, 139] were several models that
were fenestrated to improve bonding (Figs. 10−12). The true mesh trays [11,
12, 16, 44, 45, 47, 93] either were constructed from radiographs and impressions
of the stumps (Fig. 13) or were prefabricated in a range of shapes and sizes
(Fig. 14). Besides fixation with wires or screws, the mesh trays required prolonged intermaxillary fixation.

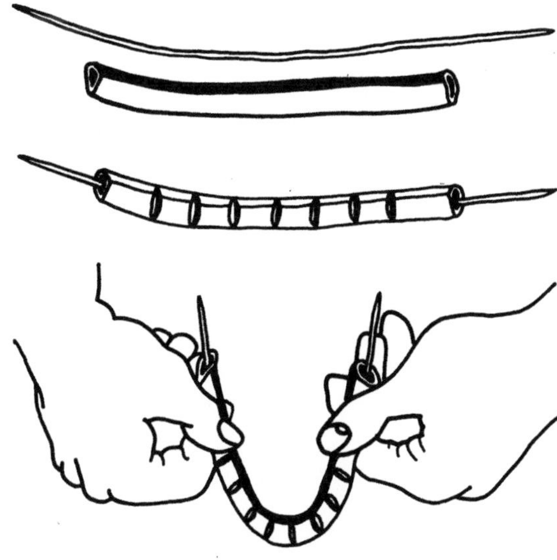

Fig. 1. Fixation of a bone graft
with a Kirschner wire: A rib graft
is made flexible by notching and
is bent to the desired shape over
1 or 2 Kirschner wires, whose ends
are anchored in the mandibular
stumps. (After MILLARD et al. [65])

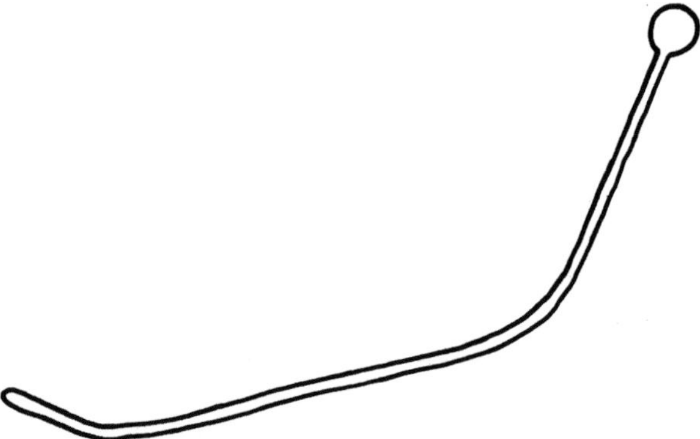

Fig. 2. Rod surmounted by a ball to replace the condylar head for alloplastic reconstruction following hemimandibulectomy. (After ANDERSON [5])

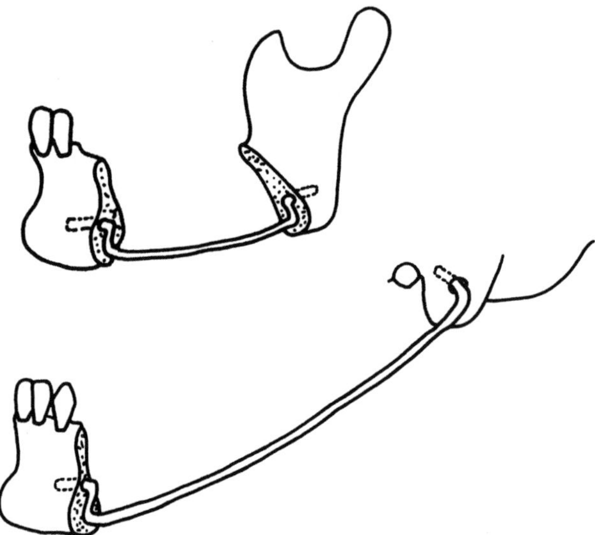

Fig. 3. Stabilization of the mandibular stump after hemimandibulectomy with a Kirschner wire bent at right angles and inserted into the mastoid to create an articular hinge. (After UPADHAYA et al. [136])

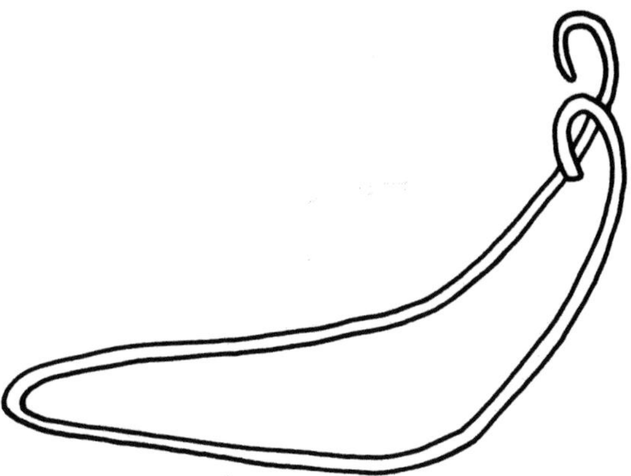

Fig. 4. The ends of a Kirschner wire are bent into loops and seated into the glenoid fossae for total reconstruction of the mandible. (After DeLathouwer et al. [55])

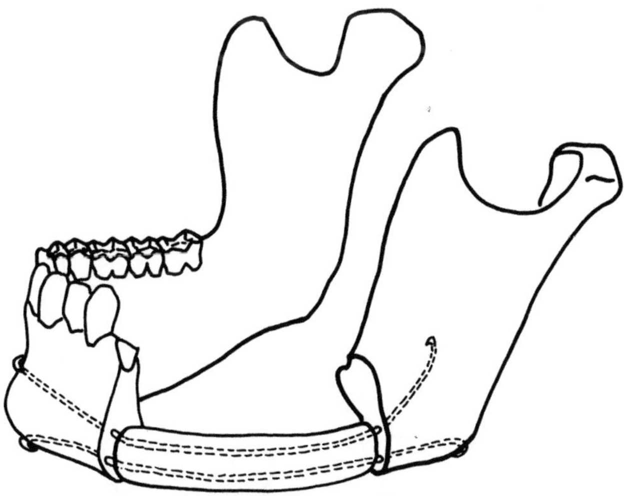

Fig. 5. A piece of silastic can be interposed to maintain separation of the mandibular stumps despite bone resorption around the rod ends. (After McQuarrie [63])

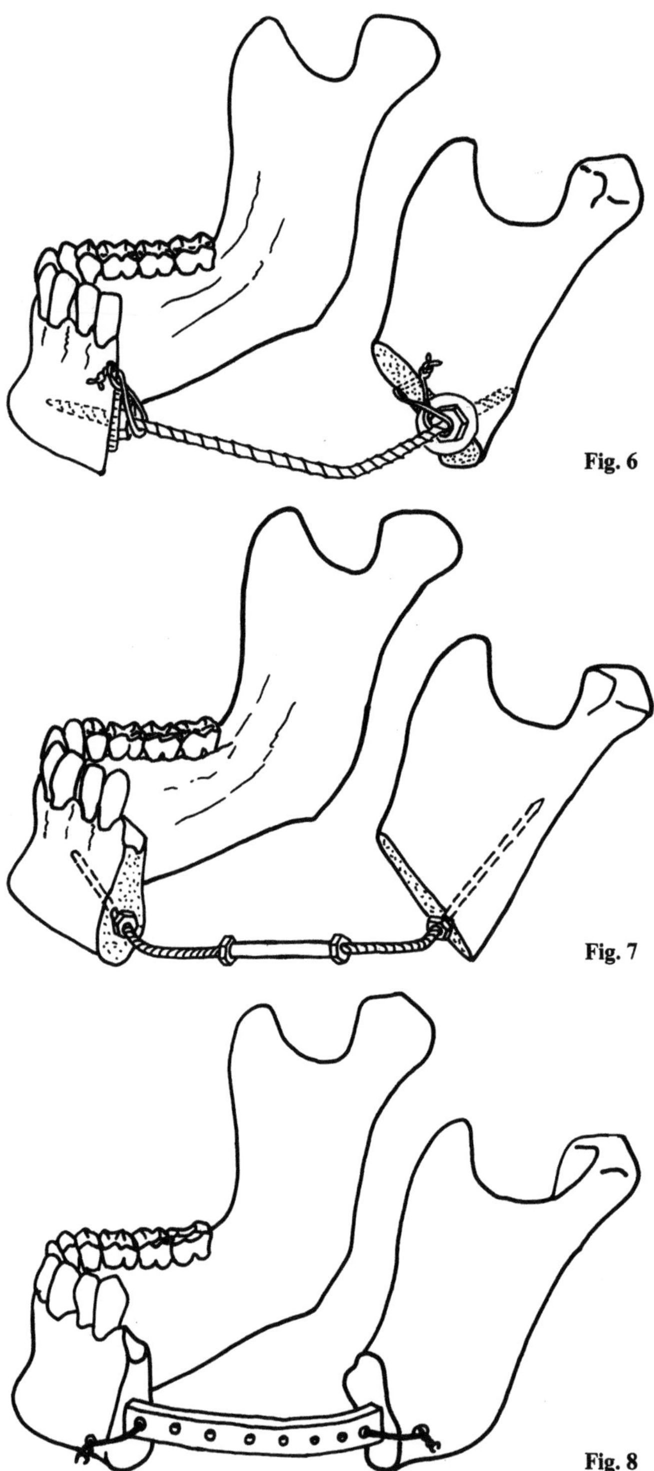

Fig. 6

Fig. 7

Fig. 8

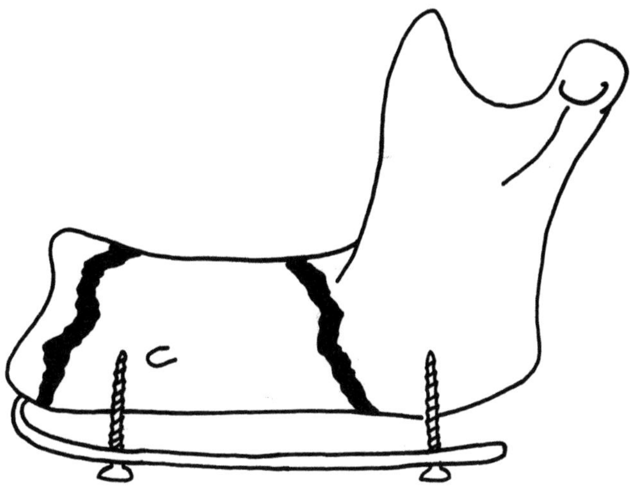

Fig. 9. External fixation with transcutaneous screws that are interconnected by a thick wire bent to the desired shape. (After PICKERILL [83])

Fig. 6. Nuts and washers on the threaded rod keep the ends from penetrating too deeply into the mandibular stumps. (After MLADICK et al. [66])

Fig. 7. Rod with a special mechanism for length adjustment in situ. (After MASSON [62])

Fig. 8. Vitallium rod, 6 or 9 cm long, 6 mm wide, 2 mm thick, whose sharpened ends are impacted into the cancellous bone and secured with wire ligatures through holes 1 mm in diameter spaced 1 cm apart (After SKALOUD [124])

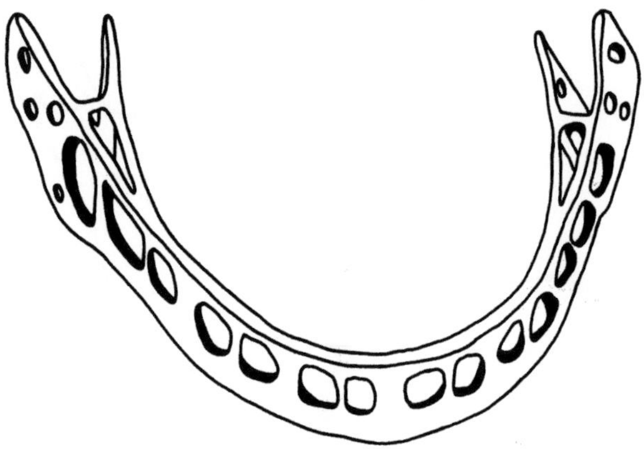

Fig. 10. Fenestrated vitallium mandibular implant. (After WINTER et al. [139])

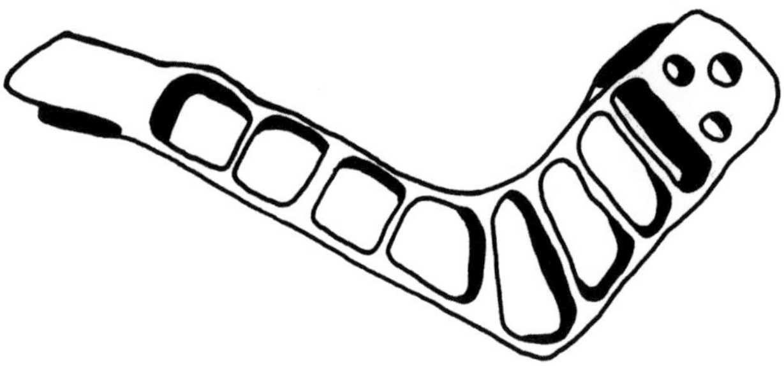

Fig. 11. Fenestrated vitallium mandibular implant. (After FREEMAN [40])

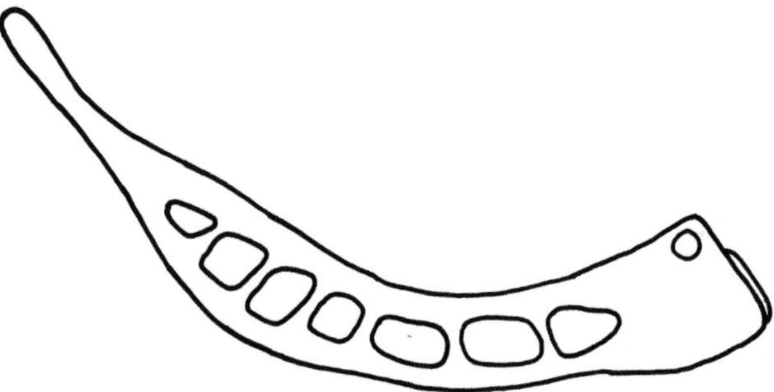

Fig. 12. Fenestrated free-end mandibular implant. (After KLEITSCH [52])

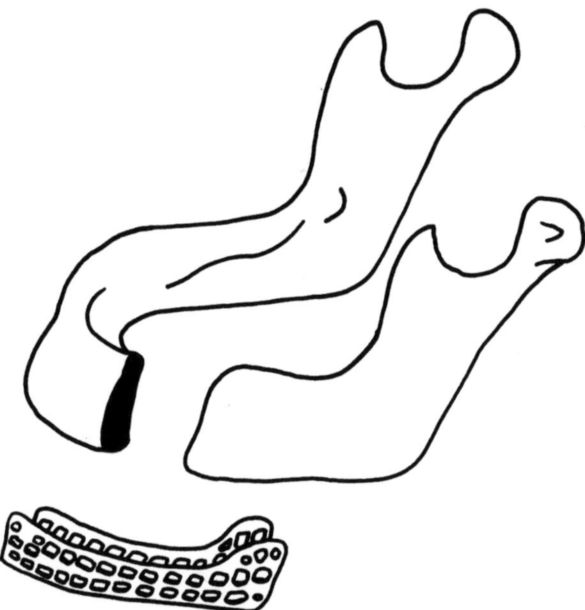

Fig. 13. Metallic mesh tray custom-fabricated from roentgenograms and models of the mandibular stumps. (After BROWN [16])

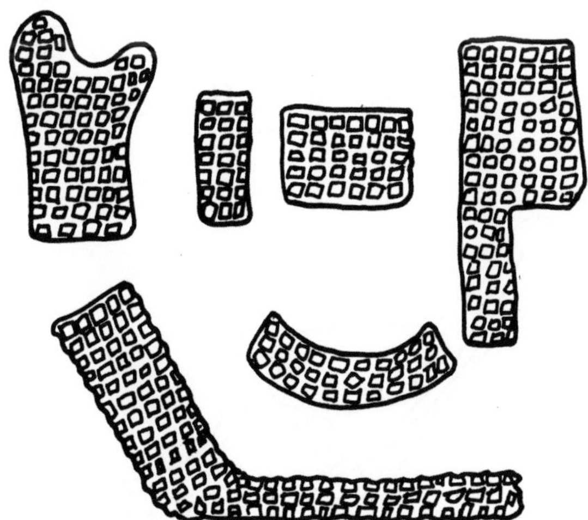

Fig. 14. Set of metallic mesh trays prefabricated in various sizes. (After HAHN and CORGILL [45])

The first *metallic prostheses* (Figs. 15 and 16, see also Figs. 10–12) for bridging large mandibular defects usually had to be removed early because of their bulky size [20, 24, 36, 52, 135]. This was prior to the development of improved models (Figs. 17–20). Condylar prostheses (Fig. 21) were designed for interpositional use in the treatment of ankylosis [108]. The prostheses were attached to the mandibular stump with Kirschner wires (Fig. 22), pins (Fig. 23), screws (Fig. 24, see also Figs. 18 and 19), wire ligatures, or methylmethacrylate [22, 24, 30, 52, 54]. Metal prostheses that are assembled from multiple parts (Fig. 25), have adjustable lengths (Fig. 26), or are fabricated in situ (Fig. 27), are more versatile in their applications [21, 93, 138].

Metal plates for securing a bone graft at both ends (Fig. 28) or for bridging across the graft (Fig. 29) were utilized in various designs, and many were prefabricated (Figs. 30 and 31) [10, 23, 25, 58]. Because of the frequent need to adapt the implant to the shape of the mandibular stumps ([59], Fig. 32), increased interest in recent years has focused on the use of plates that are bendable in all directions (Figs. 33 and 34) [7, 25, 90, 99].

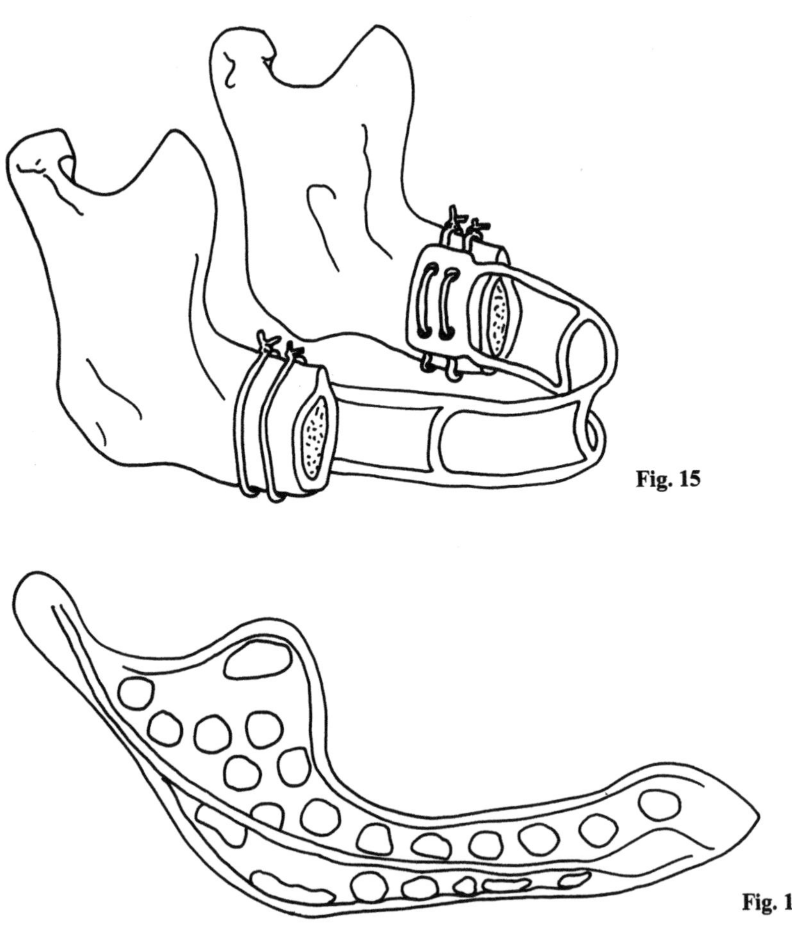

Fig. 15

Fig. 16

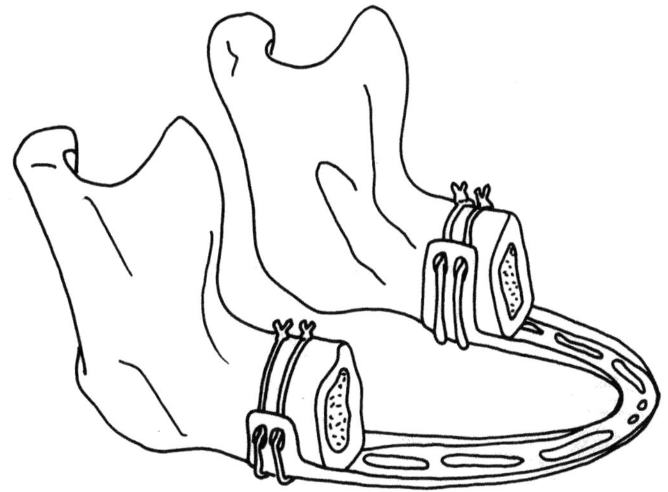

Fig. 17. Narrow mandibular implant for bridging anterior defects. (After TARNAI [135])

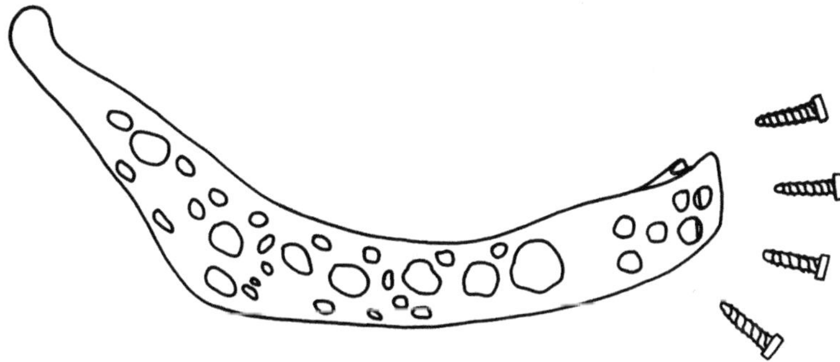

Fig. 18. Free-end mandibular implant designed for attachment with screws. (After CONLEY [24])

Fig. 15. A mandibular implant that is too wide can cause decubitus ulcers, especially in the chin area. (After TARNEI [135])

Fig. 16. Fenestrated free-end mandibular implant that imitates the shape of the mandible. (After FLINCHBAUGH [36])

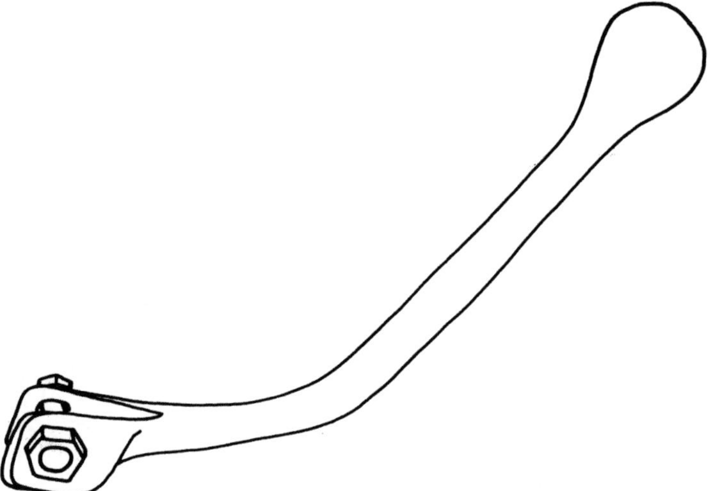

Fig. 19. Free-end mandibular implant designed for attachment with a bolt and nut. (After KLEITSCH [52])

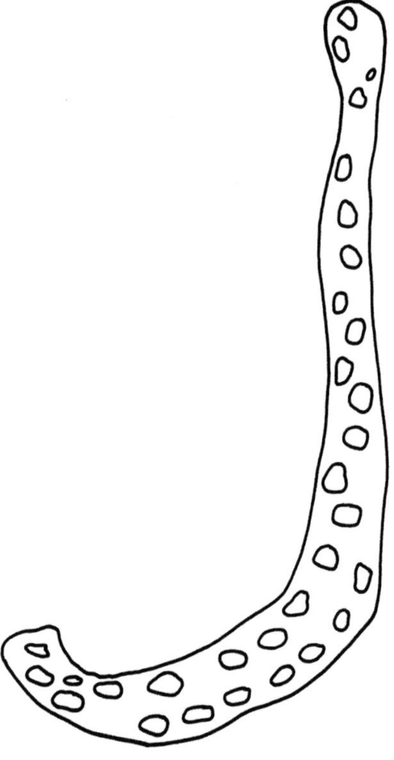

Fig. 20. Fenestrated free-end mandibular implant. (After CASTIGLIANO and GROSS [20])

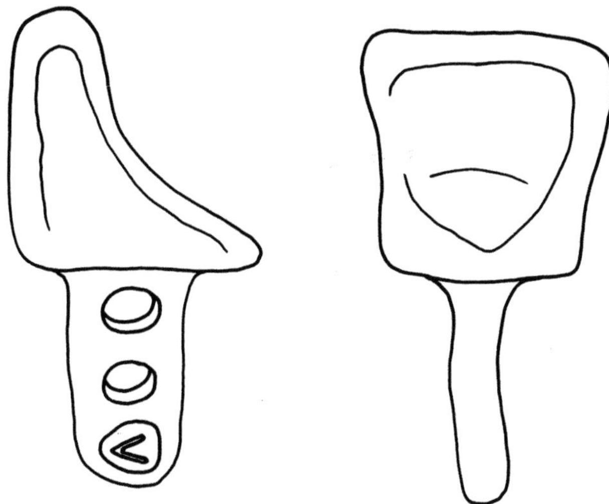

Fig. 21. Interpositional condylar prosthesis for ankylosis operations. (After SILVER et al. [123])

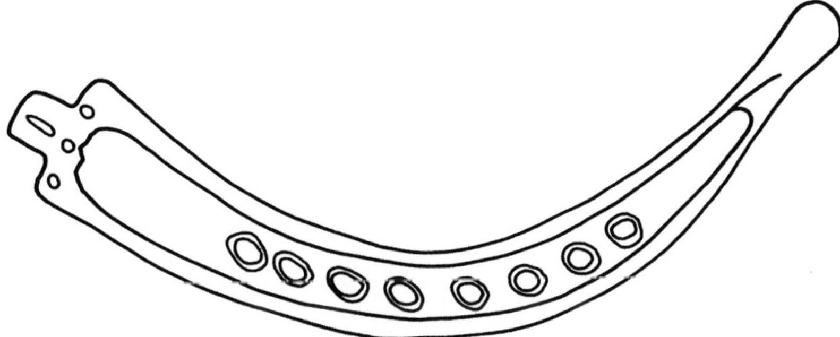

Fig. 22. Free-end mandibular implant designed for impaction into the cancellous bone and transcortical fixation with transverse Kirschner wires. (After LANE et al. [54])

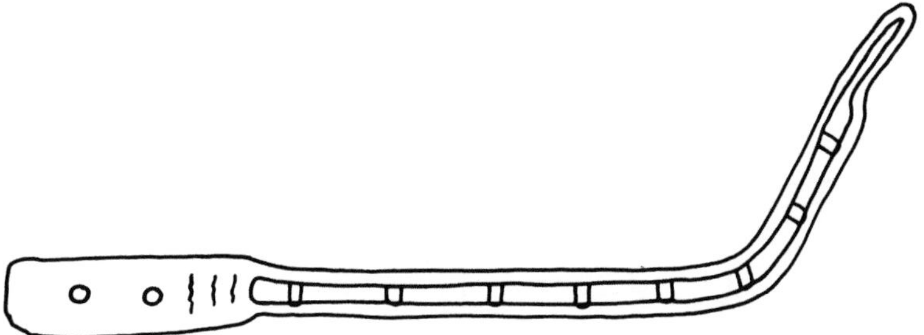

Fig. 23. Free-end mandibular implant designed for attachment with transverse pins. (After COOK [30])

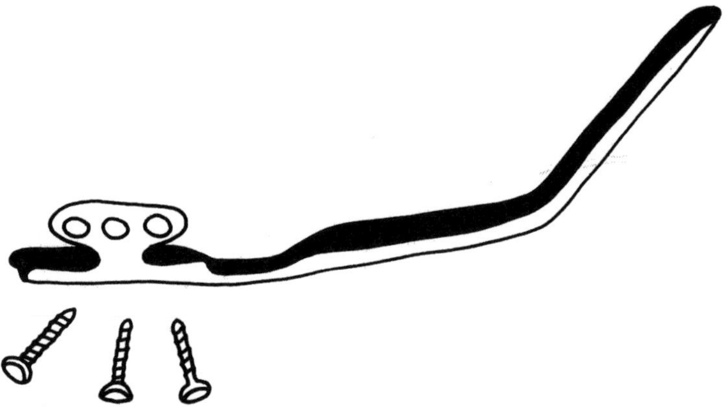

Fig. 24. Metallic trough screws to the mandibular stump, provides support for bone graft material. (After CERNEA et al. [22])

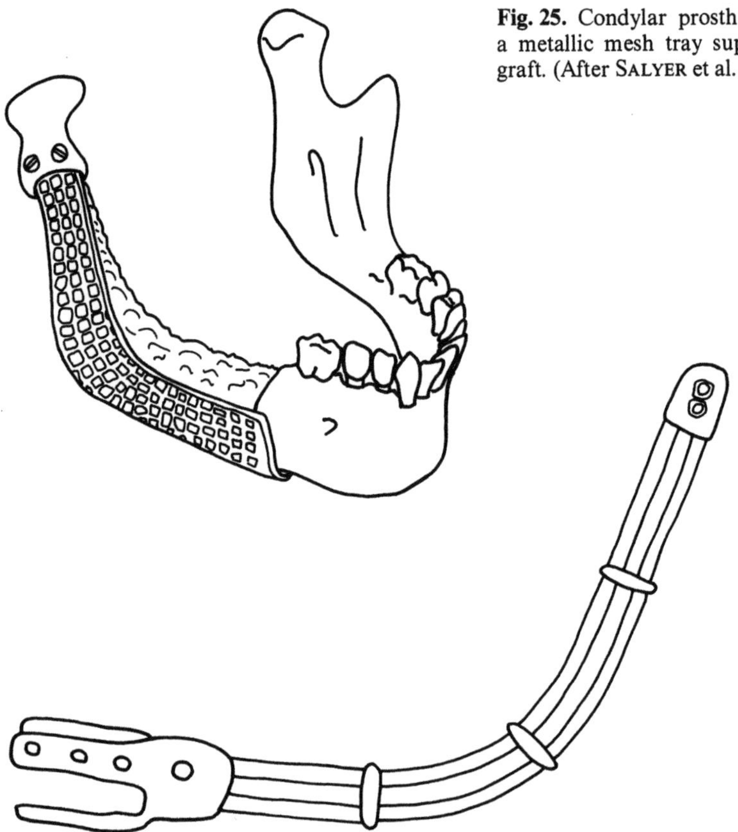

Fig. 25. Condylar prosthesis attached to a metallic mesh tray supporting a bone graft. (After SALYER et al. [93])

Fig. 26. Free-end mandibular implant that attaches to the mandibular stump. The horizontal and vertical limbs are somewhat adjustable. (After CATANIA et al. [21])

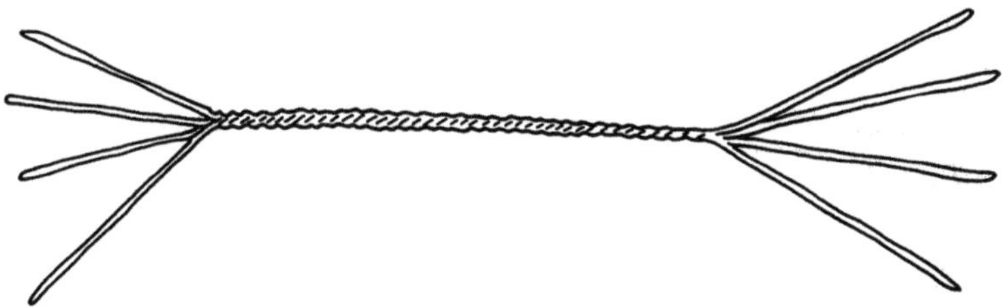

Fig. 27. Stabilization of the mandibular stumps with four wires twisted together. The free ends of the wires are anchored in the bone. (After WILSON and TOWERS [138])

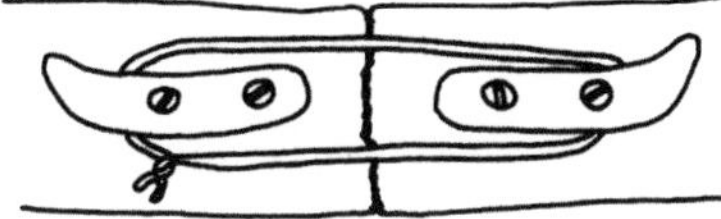

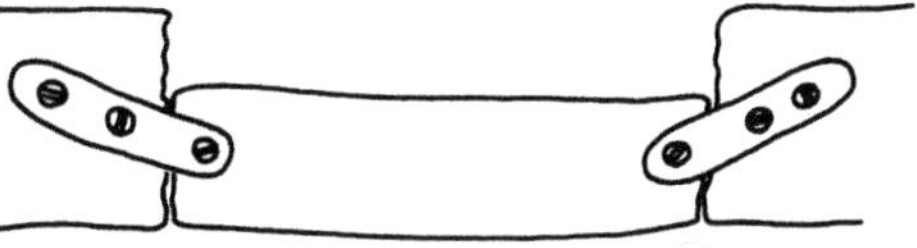

Fig. 28. Small metal plates for anchoring a bone graft to the mandibular stumps. (After COLE [23])

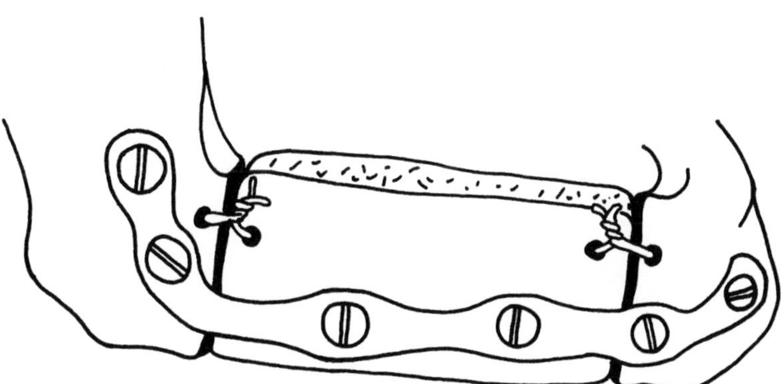

Fig. 29. Mandibular plate for securing a bone graft. The plate bridges the whole defect and stabilizes the mandibular stumps. (After CONLEY [25])

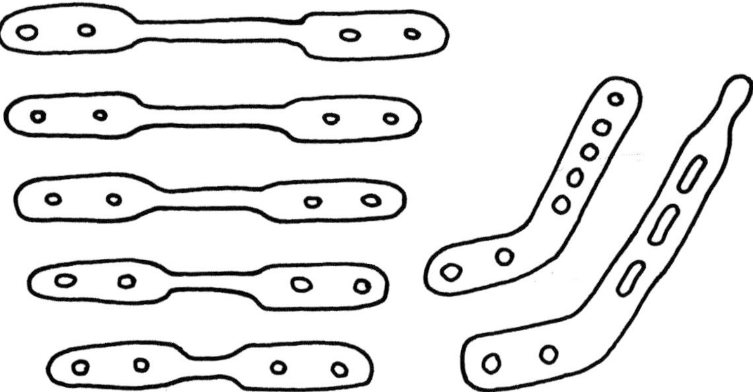

Fig. 30. Set of titanium plates that are bolted to the mandible. (After BOWERMAN and CONROY [10])

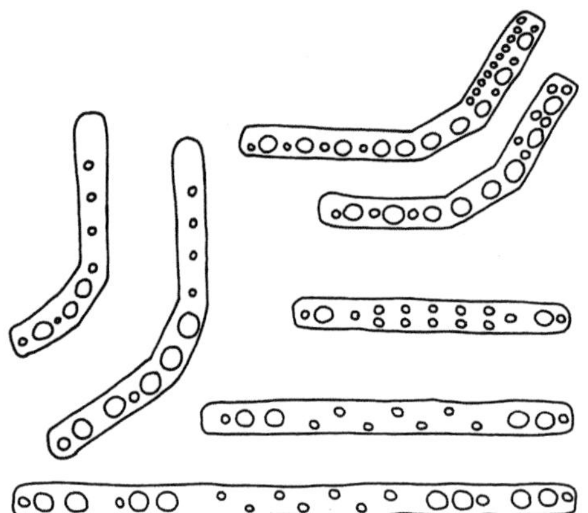

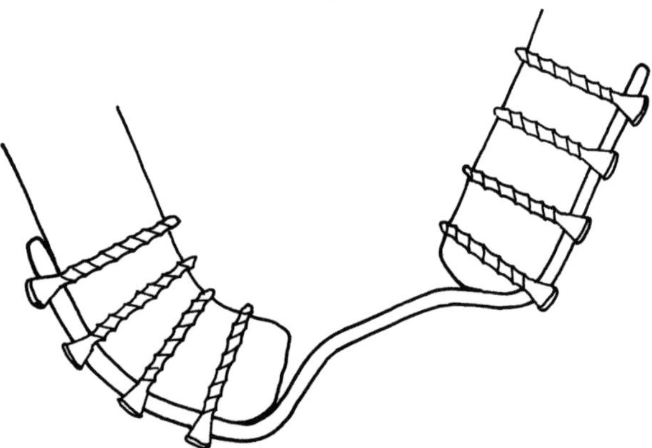

Fig. 31. Set of straight and angled plates that attach to the mandible with self-tapping screws. (After LUHR [58])

Fig. 32. The portion of the plate spanning the defect is undercontoured lingually to remove pressure from overlying soft tissues. A new plate has to be applied for secondary bone grafting. (After LUHR [59])

16

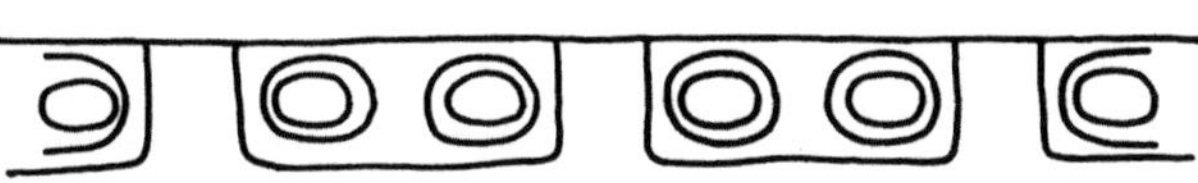

Fig. 33. Malleable metal band to which small 2-hole plates are attached for fixation to the bone. (After SCHMELZLE and SCHWENZER [99])

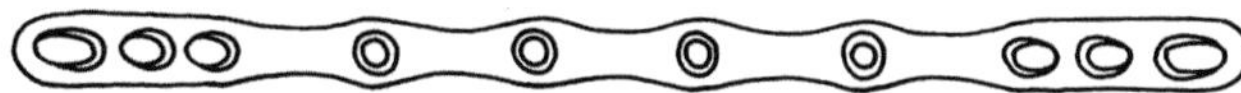

Fig. 34. This plate is bendable in all directions owing to the tapered areas between the holes. (After CONLEY [25], BECKER and MACHTENS [7], REUTHER and HAUSAMEN [90])

The *implants of today* are largely a product of biomechanical and histomorphologic research by the Swiss Association for the Study of Internal Fixation founded in 1958 by MÜLLER, ALLGÖWER, BANDI, SCHNEIDER, and WILLENEGGER [2, 3, 69−71, 81, 96−98], and of the debate sparked by this research vis-a-vis traditional implant designs (Figs. 1−34).

The problems surrounding internal fixations of the mandible are unique [100, 104, 107, 129]. The unfavorable lever arm conditions with a short force arm (vertical ramus) and a long load arm (horizontal ramus), and the consequent presence of a tension side (alveolar process) and a pressure side (mandibular border), make it difficult to achieve a functionally stable fixation in that region. Moreover, anatomic constraints allow a plate to be attached on the basal, pressure side of the mandible but not on the alveolar, tension side due to the presence of the tooth roots and nerve canal.

2 Evaluation of Preexisting Methods

The main disadvantages of the defect-bridging implants described in the literature are listed below:

Wire Ligature
- Useful only in conjunction with a bone graft
- Lack of functional stability
- Lack of functional load stimulus during intermaxillary fixation (disuse atrophy)
- Danger of infection during mobilization (infectious resorption)

Kirschner Wires and Rods
- Lack of functional stability
- Resorption at the rod ends, loosening, and dislodgment
- Initial placement unfavorable for secondary bone grafting, hence also unsuitable for temporary bridging

External Fixation
- Inconvenient for the patient
- Incites local, chronic inflammatory changes and cannot remain in place for long

Mesh Trays
- Lack of functional stability due to poor seating of the screw heads in the thin implant and poor load-bearing capacity
- Large surface area hinders bone graft revascularization and may impinge on skin and mucosa
- Tissue growth around the meshwork makes removal difficult

Metal Prostheses and Metal Plates
- Oversize implants create pressure sites and interfere with bone graft revascularization
- Fixation with wire ligatures, Kirschner wires, bolts, and self-tapping screws may not be functionally stable
- Many implants are not sufficiently adjustable, i.e., lack universal adaptability
- Holes too far apart for optimum anchorage in a minimum of space

MILLARD, in 1964, illustrated the discrepancy between the many reports of mandibular reconstructions and the relatively few reports of success by relating the ordeal of a corporal who by 1952 had undergone 21 skin flap operations and 8 bone grafts since his injury in 1944 [64]. The major cause of the failures described to date [6, 9, 12, 45] has been lack of functional stability. This has made it necessary to remove implants prematurely, often during the first 6–12 months [9, 42], and has led to serious consequences due to the proximity of the glenoid fossa to the skull base, as illustrated by one case where a loose prosthesis migrated into the cranial cavity (Obwegeser 1979, personal communication). Some of the disadvantages of the various methods are considered below.

Kirschner wires and rods do not provide a functionally stable fixation of the mandibular stumps. Soon after implantation resorption occurs around the ends of the rod, followed by loosening and expulsion. Hence this mode of fixation is also unsuitable for the temporary briding of defects [19, 42].

External fixation is most appropriate in patients who have coexisting soft-tissue defects. The inconvenience to the patient and the occurrence of chronic inflammatory changes around the pin sites limit the duration of use [18].

The U-shaped metallic *mesh trays* are frequently used with bone grafts, but the poor seating of the screw heads in the hole of the thin tray and its proneness to deformation make it unsuitable for the functionally stable bridging of defects — hence the need for concurrent intermaxillary fixation. The main function of the mesh tray is to support transplanted cancellous bone. Its U shape hinders remodeling of the mandible. Despite its meshwork structure, the implant interferes with bone graft revascularization. Its large size may cause pressure lesions on the overlying skin and mucosa. After the cancellous bone graft has healed, tissue growth around the framework makes it very difficult to remove [12, 33, 44, 45, 56, 122, 127].

Metal prostheses and metal plates that mimic the anatomic shape of the mandibular segment to be replaced lead to pressure sites and hinder the revascularization of grafted bone. Because many implants are not bendable, they cannot be used in all patients. Models that are tapered between holes to improve their malleability have their holes spaced too far apart to provide optimum anchorage in a minimum of space. The implants are attached to the bone with self-tapping screws; this is less desirable than using an instrument set specifically designed for drilling and tapping the bone. Free-end prostheses cannot all be fixed in a functionally stable manner. The design of most prosthetic condyles is limited to a simple spherical shape [20, 26, 37, 40, 52, 67, 135, 139].

3 Statement of Problem

Our main challenge was to achieve a stable fixation of the reconstructed mandible consistent with the requirements of early postoperative function. For this purpose we had to create a *new implant design* oriented toward the peculiar mechanical characteristics of the mandible.

The following problems had to be addressed:

Development of Implants
acceptable in terms of:
− clinical requirements
− functional stability (immediate mobilization)
− the biomechanical characteristics of the mandible

Testing the Implants in Laboratory Animals
− development of an acceptable animal model
− scope of animal experimentation
− achievement of functional stability
− functional stability vs. extent of mandibular defect
− applicability of the implants
− ways of improving the implants
− technique of insertion
− surgical approach
− tissue compatibility
− resistance to fracture
− function of condylar head
− reaction of contralateral joint
− possibility and method of placement of abutments
− stability of the abutment anchorage
− danger of open communication with the oral cavity
− epithelial margin around the abutment
− ease of implant removal.

Once we had designed the implants, it remained to test and improve them in clinically oriented animal experiments.

The clinical requirements of the implants are listed below:

− functionally stable bridging of defects without intermaxillary fixation
− temporary or definitive fixation of the mandibular stumps in the anatomically correct position
− holes spaced close together for optimum fixation in a minimum amount of space
− large enough to resist fracture
− small enough to permit revascularization of grafted bone and avoid pressure on overlying skin and mucosa

- option for primary or secondary bone grafting
- bendable in all directions
- replacement of mandibular condyle
- means for denture fixation
- uncomplicated removal.

There was need to find a suitable *animal model* in which the clinical requirements could be properly tested. In so doing, it was necessary to define clinical and morphologic criteria by which the functional performance of the reconstructed mandible could be objectively assessed.

Our main goal was to achieve *functional stability* that would obviate the need for intermaxillary fixation once the mandibular arch and joint had been reconstructed. In experimental animals, normal feeding provides the best test of stability under loading and goes beyond simple testing of exercise stability. The *extent of the defect* had to be such that it would constitute a stringent test of the functional stability of the reconstruction.

Areas of major concern were the *universal adaptability of the implants* (e.g., their malleability and resistance to fracture when fitted to the mandible), improvement of the implants, the usefulness of the instrument set, and questions of *insertion technique* (e.g., the number of screws needed for a functionally stable anchorage, the length of the prosthetic stem).

We wished also to compare the extraoral approach with the combined intra-/extraoral approach in order to identify the *best surgical approach* in terms of the risk of infection.

To establish the duration of the experimental study, we conducted *preliminary experiments* to determine the point in the postoperative course when the final result could be definitively assessed on the basis of bone remodeling.

In the longer term we were interested in assessing the *tissue compatibility* of the implants and the *reaction of the implant bed,* especially the influence of stable and unstable conditions and the effect of healthy and damaged bony and soft tissues in the implant environment.

In the region of the replaced condylar head, we wished to assess the *function of the joint* in the live animal, testing its passive mobility grossly after necropsy and assessing microscopically the reactions of the articular fossa and contralateral joint.

In the region of the *abutment,* our questions centered on the possibility of anchoring the abutment directly to the reconstruction plate without prior bone grafting, and on the stability of the anchorage. We were also interested in the effect of the tissue surrounding the abutment in cases of *transmucosal, transalveolar,* and *transosseous* placement of the abutment. We were particularly concerned about the possibility of *infection* and its spread from the oral cavity along the abutment post and anchoring element to the plate and to the condylar head of the prosthesis.

Also in connection with the abutment, we wished to investigate the *epithelial investment* of the post and the possibility and extent of epithelial downgrowth.

A final area of concern was the *ease of removal* of the implants, which has an important bearing on their clinical use.

To address all the questions of interest, it was necessary to conduct *comparative studies* in which the experimental animals were divided into groups:

- with and without the *number of screws* necessary for a functionally stable fixation, to determine the necessary extent of the anchorage;
- with and without an *abutment* projecting freely into the oral cavity, to assess its potential as a portal for infection;
- with *transmucosal, transalveolar, and transosseous* placement of the abutment, to establish the most favorable insertion technique;
- with an extraoral *approach* and with a combined intra-/extraoral approach, to evaluate the risk of infection associated with opening of the unsterile oral cavity during the operation;
- with and without *periosteal stripping* in the area of the alveolar ridge, to assess the viability of bone stumps denuded of periosteum;
- with and without the cutting of a *skin flap*, to observe the effect of blood flow impairment on the soft-tissue coverage of the plate;
- animals with 3−4 months' *survival time* and animals surviving 3 years, to study the effects of prolonged loading.

Part I: Experimental Studies

Materials and Methods

1 Implants

The development of our implants (Figs. 35–46) was based upon published criticisms of the implants described earlier (see list on p. 17) and on discoveries made during the clinical reconstruction of mandibular defects (see list on p. 19). Experience since 1973 with the "Eccentric Dynamic Compression Plate" [100, 101, 104, 105, 107] shows that the use of this device should be limited to the internal fixation of less severe mandibular defects.

The basic features of the newly developed implants are as follows:

Mandibular Reconstruction Plate

Design: 2.7 mm × 7.8 mm cross-section
Minimal hole spacing (8 mm)
Composed of 6-mm segments separated by U-shaped notches 2 mm wide by 1.5 mm deep
Bidirectional DC holes
Used with 2.7-mm spherical-head cortex screws (may be inserted obliquely) and with 3.5-mm cortex screws with the spherical head of the 2.7 screw

Models: Straight model: 6–24 holes
Prebent model: right and left mandibular angle in three sizes
Total mandible in three sizes

Pliers: 1 Bending pliers for bending on the flat
2 Bending pliers for edgewise bending and for twisting
1 Cutting pliers for shortening the plate

Condylar Prosthesis

Design: Head, neck, stem. Stem offset 4.2 mm from axis of head and neck; vertical and horizontal limbs meet at 125° angle

Head: Bispherical transverse oval 9 × 13.5 mm, radii 3.7 mm and 10 mm, neck 11 mm, right and left models in 3 sizes (vertical limb 40 mm with 2 DC holes, 45 and 50 mm with 3 DC holes)

Neck: 11 mm long with 7 × 11-mm baseplate bearing spike 4 mm long by 2.3 mm in diameter

Stem: Cross-section 2.5 mm × 7.8 mm; U-shaped notches 2 mm wide by 1.5 mm deep; horizontal limb 24 mm long with 3 round holes

Right and left models in 3 sizes:
Vertical limb in lengths of 40 mm (2 DC holes), 45 and 50 mm (3 DC holes)

Reconstruction Plate with Condylar Head

Design: Head, stem with vertical and horizontal limbs angled 125°

Head: Bispherical transverse oval 9 × 13.5 mm, radii 3.7 mm and 10 mm

Stem: Cross-section 2.7 mm × 7.8 mm
          Holes spaced 8 mm apart
          Composed of 6-mm segments separated by U-shaped notches 2 mm wide and 1.5 mm
          deep
          Bidirectional DC holes
          Used with 2.7-mm spherical-head cortex screws

Right and left models in 3 sizes:
          Vertical limb 50, 55, and 60 mm
          Horizontal limb 128, 144, and 160 mm

Anchoring Element for Abutments

Dimensions: 10 mm × 10 mm × 5 mm

Anchorage: Screw with M2 metal thread and spherical head of 2.7-mm screw

Abutment lengths: 9, 11, 13, and 17 mm

1.1 Mandibular Reconstruction Plate

In 1973 we began working with the manufacturer, Dr. R. Mathys, to develop a
reconstruction plate for the bridging of mandibular defects. Initially the plate
was patterned after the ASIF dynamic compression plate for 4.5-mm screws [2,
3, 8] and later after the ASIF clavicular plate. We have used the mandibular
reconstruction plate in its present form and dimensions (Fig. 35) since 1976
[113, 115].

All implants are fabricated from stainless steel (DIN No. 4435). The plate is
2.7 mm thick, 7.8 mm wide, and has an arched cross-section. The holes are
spaced 8 mm apart. The individual plate segments are 6 mm in length. The
plate attaches to the mandible with 2.7-mm cortex screws; a corresponding tap
is used to prethread the drill holes in the bone. U-shaped notches 2 mm wide

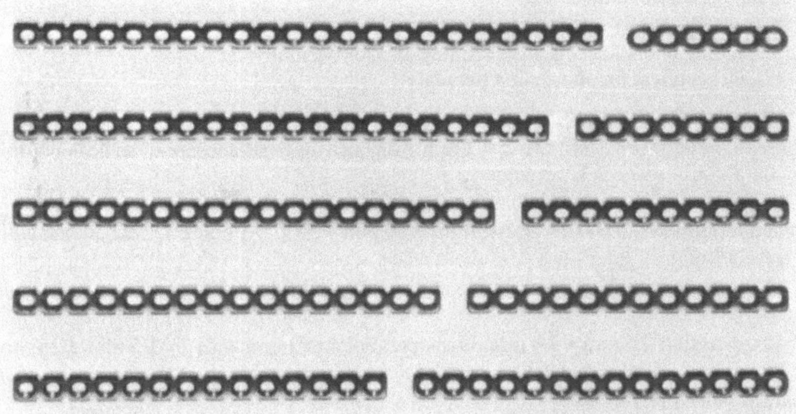

Fig. 35. The three-dimensionally bendable reconstruction plate (3-DBRP) is produced in
various lengths (6, 8, 10, . . . , 24 holes). The holes are spaced closely together, and the plate
edges are notched between the holes. The plates can be shortened as needed by cutting them
at the notches with plate cutting pliers

24

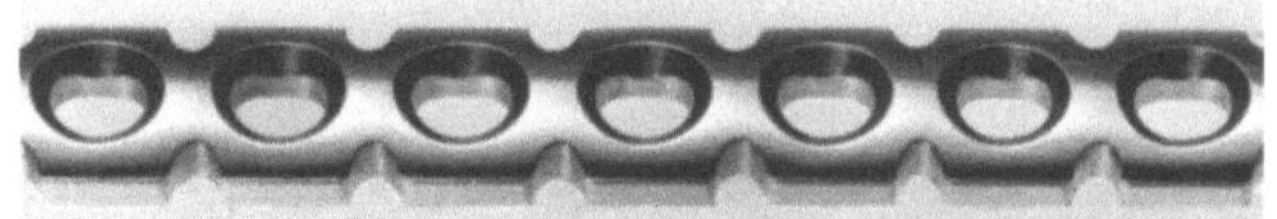

Fig. 36. The plates have bidirectional DC holes that are operative in both longitudinal directions. As the screw is driven in, its spherical head slides down along the inclined surface of the plate hole (spherical gliding principle) in one or the other longitudinal direction, depending on the placement of the eccentric drill hole. The edges of the plate are notched between adjacent plate holes

are spaced at regular intervals along the edges of the plate, between adjacent pairs of holes (Fig. 36). These notches enable the plate to be bent edgewise as well as on the flat. Edgewise bending is done with the aid of two specially designed pliers ([115], see also Fig. 40), and a plate that has been angled in this fashion can be restraightened if desired. The presence of the notches gives the plate a roughly uniform cross-section throughout. Thus the holes do not create points of weakness, and the plate bends at the level of the notches rather than at the holes, even when it is bent on the flat. As a result, the reconstruction plate is adjustable not just in two directions on one plane but in all three spatial directions (Three Dimensionally Bendable Reconstruction Plate, 3-DBRP). DCP holes[1] are designed to produce compression across the fracture site and hence are directed toward the center of the plate. The development of two-way DC holes that function bidirectionally (Fig. 36) enables compression to be exerted in both longitudinal directions [115].

These holes also ensure a solid seating of the screw head in the plate hole, even when the screw is inserted obliquely. Besides the straight plates, prebent models were produced in three sizes each (Figs. 37 and 38). Already, initial reports have been published on the development and clinical use of the reconstruction plate [109, 111, 113, 115, 127, 128, 131].

We have also developed a miniaturized version of the plate (mini-reconstruction plate) for use on the maxilla and for use with 2.0-mm screws.

1.2 Condylar Prosthesis

Both cemented [123] and uncemented articular prostheses [5] owe their anchorage to frictional bonding between the stem of the prosthesis and the bone.

---

1 DCP = "Dynamic Compression Plate" [2, 3, 8]. The DC hole is based on the spherical gliding principle and is formed geometrically by the intersection of an inclined half-cylinder with a horizontal half-cylinder. As a screw is inserted, its spherical head glides down the inclined portion of the DC hole, producing a longitudinal movement of the underlying bone fragment relative to the plate. When a screw is driven into the opposing fragment, the same process takes place in the opposite direction. The result is a longitudinal displacement of both fragments toward each other, producing compression across the fracture site. Thus, the DC holes translate the vertical, downward movement of the screw heads into a horizontal displacement of the fragments.

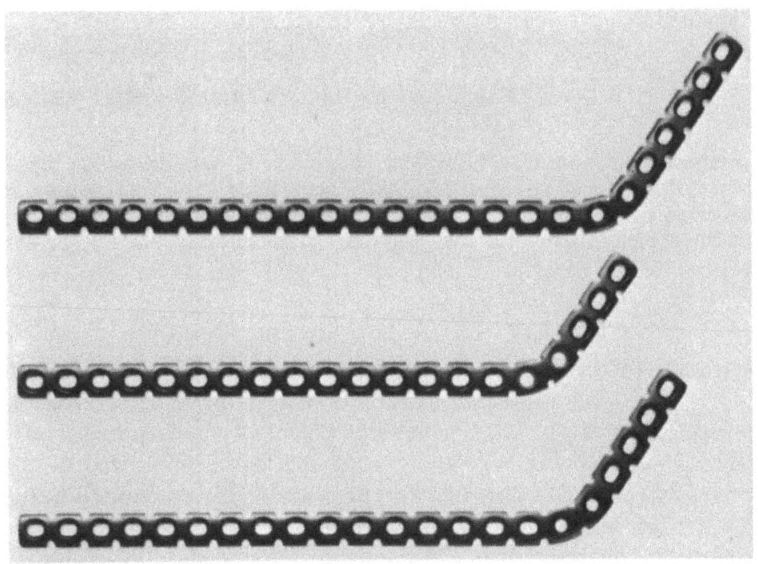

Fig. 37. Preshaped plates are manufactured in three different sizes and in right- and left-sided designs for reconstructing the hemimandible

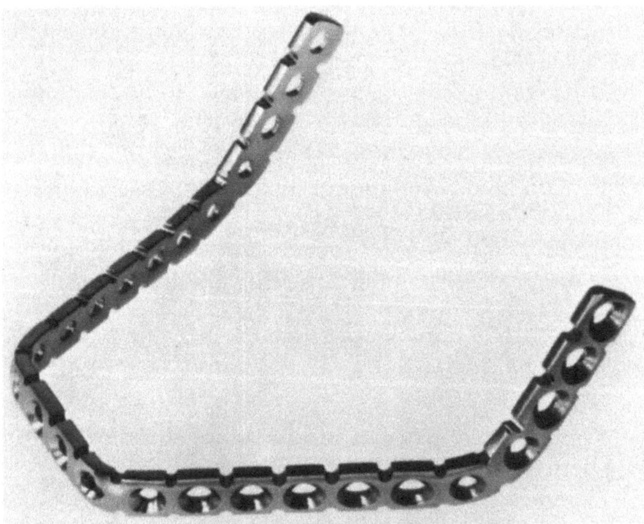

Fig. 38. Preshaped plate for reconstructing the entire mandible excluding the condylar processes

The strength of this bond can be greatly enhanced by the use of compression screws. The eccentric placement of a screw through a DC hole produces a compressive force along the screw axis. By using DC holes in conjunction with a compression surface at right angles to the stem axis (the baseplate of the neck of the prosthesis), a tensile force is also generated which presses the prosthetic stem against the bone surface. The compressive and tensile force supplement each other to maintain anchorage of the prosthesis.

Because the sites of action of the load (head of prosthesis) and the stabilization (baseplate with spike) are spaced about 10 mm apart, a load that is not strictly axial will exert a rotational force on the prosthesis. This torque can be neutralized by selecting the longest possible prosthetic stem.

Studies in cadaveric jaws showed that the following areas of the mandibular bone are most competent to withstand loads:

1. The *neck of the mandible,* in accordance with its function as a tubular bone, is most resistant to axial loading and thus makes a suitable abutment surface for the cervical baseplate of the prosthesis.
2. The thin bone of the *vertical ramus* is most resistant to bending on the sagittal plane, corresponding to the direction of pull of the attached muscles. Compression screws can create a primary stress on this plane to seat the baseplate of the prosthesis solidly against the neck of the mandible.
3. The bony *base of the mandible* possesses two thick cortical plates spaced about 10 mm apart. Screws anchored in this bone neutralize both the sagittal component of the torque, which tends to displace the prosthetic stem along the lateral surface of the vertical ramus, and also the transverse force component, which tends to raise the prosthetic stem from the bone.

The most recent design of our condylar prosthesis, as documented in 1977 [114], consists of a head, neck, and stem in right- and left-sided models. Fixation is accomplished by a spiked baseplate below the neck of the prosthesis and by the vertical and horizontal limbs of the stem. The limbs join at a 125° angle.

A large *condylar head* has a larger contact surface than a small head but is also more susceptible to dislocation. For this reason we gave the head of the prosthesis a bispherical, transverse oval shape; thus the radius on the frontal plane is larger than the radius on the sagittal plane. The small head radius offers more resistance to dislocation on the sagittal plane than does the large radius on the frontal plane. Meanwhile, dislocation on the frontal plane is opposed medially by the shape of the glenoid fossa and laterally by the retentive structures of the contralateral joint. Thus the bispherical, transverse oval shape of the condyle represents a tradeoff between maximum contact surface on the one hand, and minimum dislocation risk on the other.

The *neck* of the prosthesis is positioned atop a baseplate, which seats against the stump of the mandibular neck. A 4-mm-long spike at the center of the baseplate is impacted into the cancellous bone of the articular process.

The *prosthetic stem* can be bent edgewise owing to the presence of U-shaped notches along its edges (analogous to the reconstruction plate). The vertical limb has 2 or 3 DC holes, depending on the model, and comes in 40-, 45-, or 50-

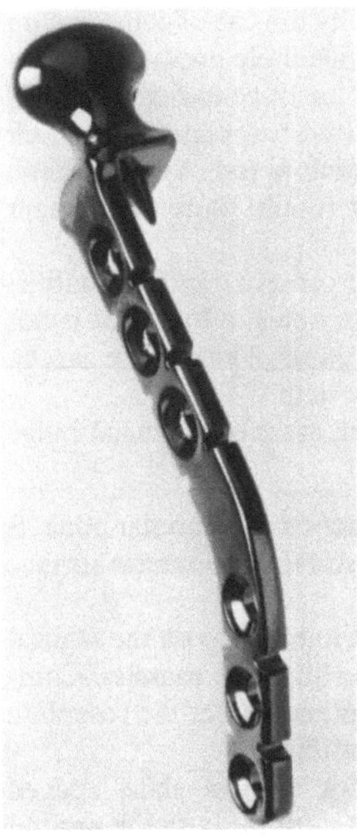

Fig. 39. The condylar prosthesis consists of a head, neck, and stem. The baseplate with spike is compressed against the bony neck stump by means of the 3 DC holes in the vertical limb. The implant is additionally secured to the base of the mandible through the holes in the horizontal limb

mm lengths. Driving screws into the DC holes has the effect of pressing the baseplate against the articular process. The lower limb of the prosthesis has a total of three round holes, which accept lag screws. These screws and the screws in the DC holes produce the static tensile forces perpendicular to the long axis of the bone.

Besides a paper on the development and experimental testing of the condylar prosthesis [114], reports have already been published on initial clinical experience with these implants [109, 116, 117, 126, 132].

1.3 Reconstruction Plate with Condylar Head

The reconstruction plate with condylar head ([114], Figs. 40–42) represents a combination of the prebent mandibular reconstruction plate and the condylar prosthesis. Like the standard reconstruction plate, the reconstruction plate with condylar head can be bent or twisted in all directions with special pliers. The vertical limb comes in lengths of 50, 55, or 60 mm, and all prebent plates are angled 125°. Both right- and left-sided models are available. Initial reports on animal studies and clinical experience have been published [109, 117].

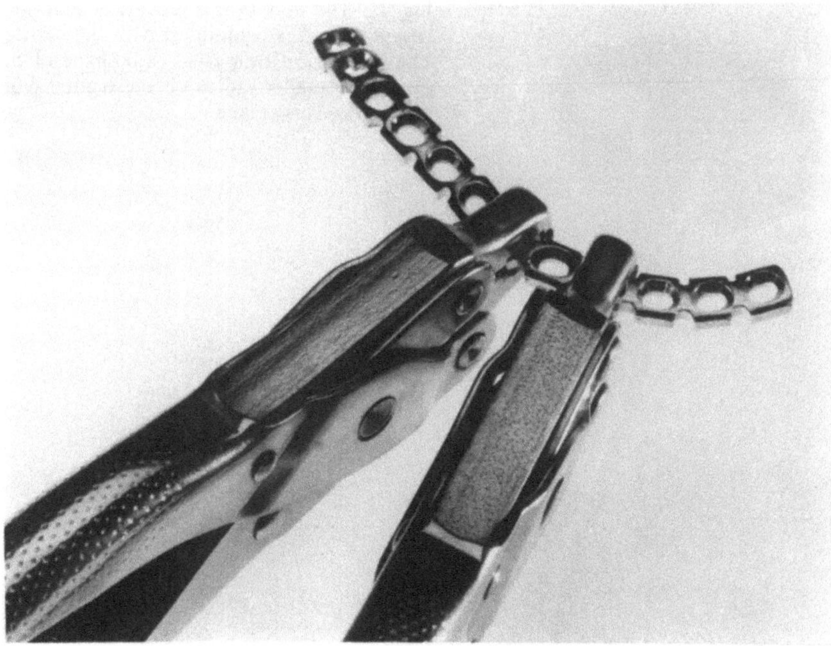

Fig. 40. The reconstruction plate is adapted to the mandible with special bending pliers, which are applied over the plate segments so that bending or twisting will occur at the U-shaped notches

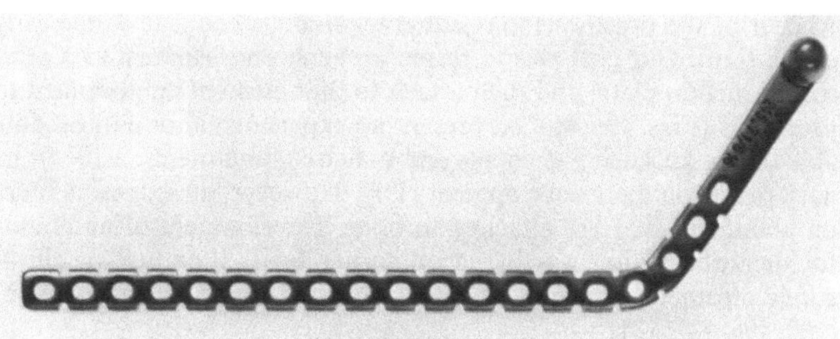

Fig. 41. Reconstruction plate with condylar head. The length of the horizontal limb enables the plate to be attached across the midline to the contralateral ramus

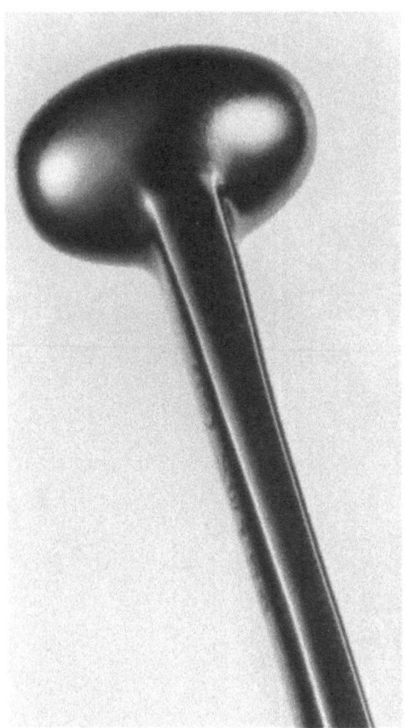

Fig. 42. The neck of this prosthesis does not have a baseplate and is continuous with the vertical limb. The bispherical transverse oval shape of the head gives it a smaller radius on the sagittal plane than on the transverse plane

1.4 Anchoring Element for Abutments

The placement of a denture to restore masticatory function is problematic after the bridging of a mandibular defect due to the absence of the alveolar crest. Anchoring the prosthesis to residual teeth alone can lead to the early loosening of the teeth. Our goal was to fasten an anchoring element to a segment of the reconstruction plate, and then attach to that element an abutment to support a prosthesis (Figs. 43–46). At present no experimental or clinical data are available on the anchoring elements and matching abutments, aside from a preliminary report on their development [114]. However, an extensive literature exists on abutments that are attached to bone. Development of an abutment system for denture fixation was based on earlier Swiss literature on the functionally stable prosthetic implant [125] and on related experimental and clinical studies [102, 106, 112, 131].

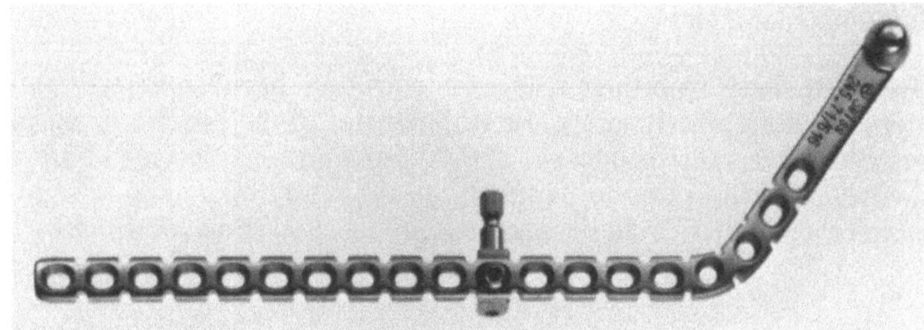

Fig. 43. Special anchoring elements were designed that screw into the holes of the reconstruction plate and provide means for attaching denture abutments

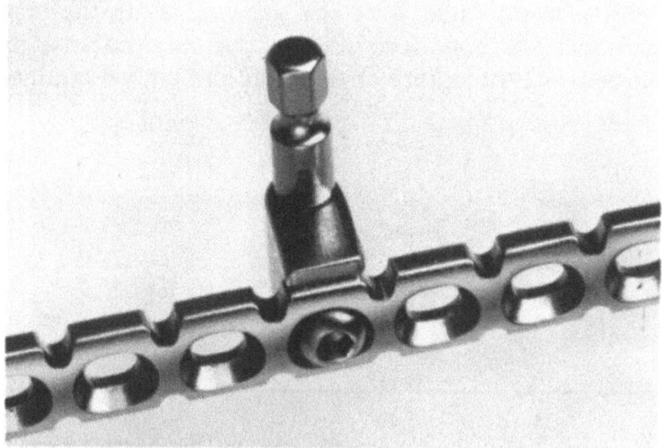

Fig. 44. Close-up view of an abutment screwed into the anchoring element. The anchoring element attaches to the plate with an ordinary 2.7-mm cortex screw

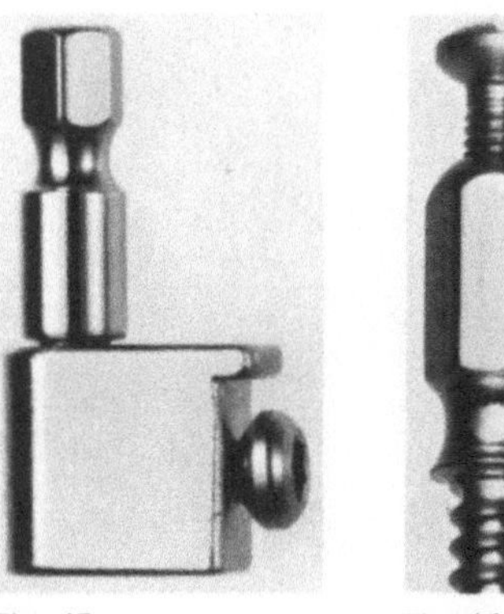

Fig. 45. The anchoring element/abutment assembly, with screw for attachment to the plate. The abutments come in various lengths and are selected according to the thickness of the tissue over the anchoring element

Fig. 46. This abutment is internally threaded to accommodate retention elements for the attachment of a denture-supporting superstructure

Fig. 45   **Fig. 46**

2 Animal Experiments

Our preliminary experiments were conducted in sheep, an animal whose grinding mastication provided a most stringest test of the prosthetic anchorage, especially under transverse loads. The experiments were designed both to test the condylar prosthesis and to establish the time after operation at which the parameters of interest could be meaningfully assessed (Figs. 47 and 48).

2.1 Experimental Animal

Choice of experimental animal: To investigate the newly developed reconstruction plates, we had to have an animal model whose masticatory function and jaw morphology approximated that of humans as closely as possible. It was our intention to test the reconstruction plates in fully mature animals as well as animals that were still growing. With the object of evaluating weight gain and new bone formation as our chief parameters, we had to operate on animals – even mature ones – that had not yet attained their full body weight.

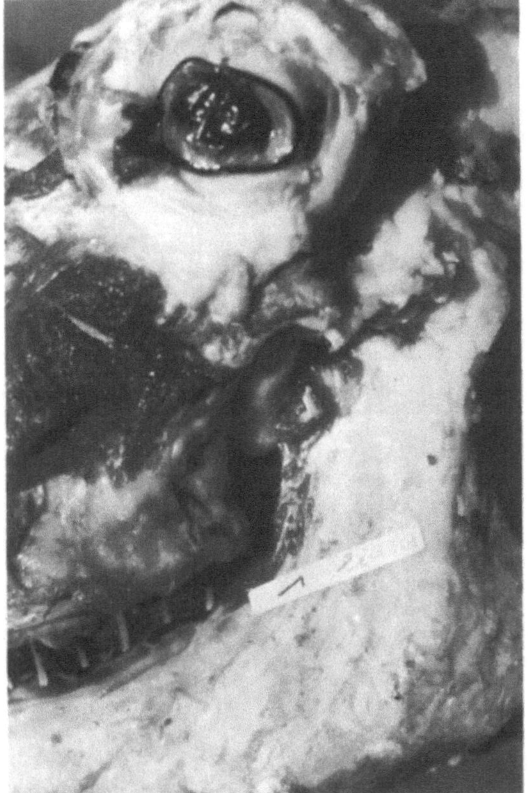

Fig. 47 a – c. Condylar prosthesis in a sheep 9 months after resection and replacement of the condyle head (animal 1). **a** The prosthesis and screw heads are covered by bone. **b** The bony deposit has been removed with a chisel to expose the prosthesis. **c** Bed of prosthesis with periosteal new bone formation along the prosthetic margins. The screw beds are invested by bone

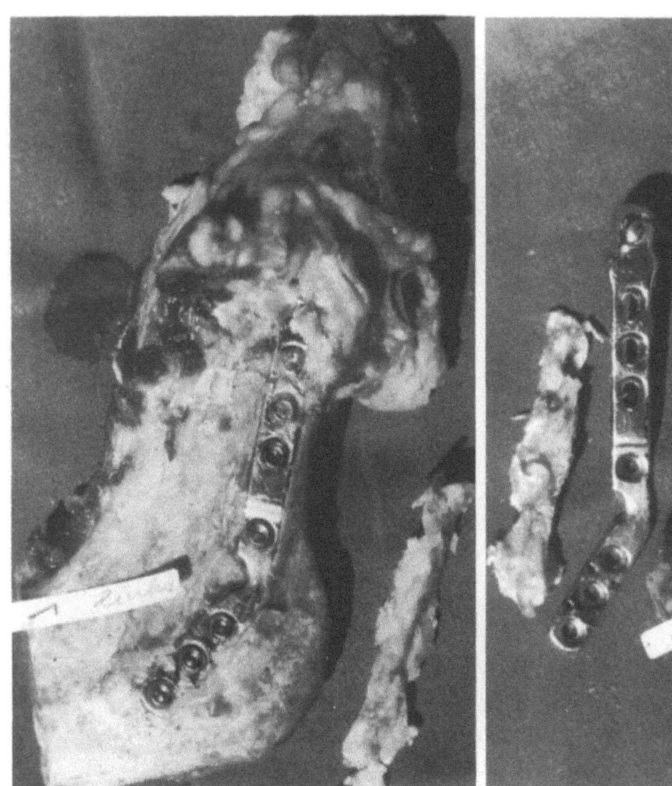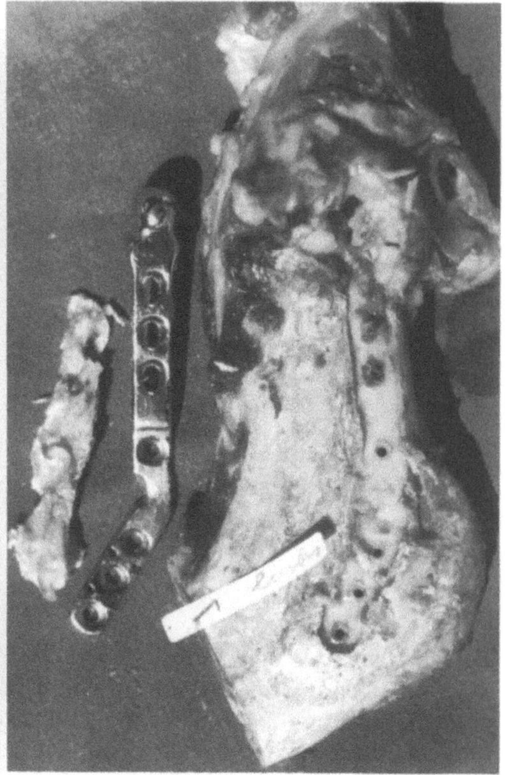

Fig. 47 b, c

Another requirement was that the size of the mandible in the adult animal approximate that in humans. The animal that best fulfilled these requirements was the 5- to 12-month-old *minipig*. We performed our experiments on a total of 44 minipigs with initial body weights of 16 to 59 kg.

Maintenance of the animals: The minipigs were housed in box stalls, with several animals per stall, and were fed dry chow (UFA Complete Feed). Antibiotic coverage consisted of premedication with spectacillin (Sandoz), 1−2 g i.v., followed by Cobiotic (Pfizer), 5 ml i.m., for 3 days.

Anesthesia (Table 1): The animals were intubated following premedication with Ketalar (Parke Davis), up to 12.5 mg/kg BW i.m., and induction with Stresnil (Cilag), 2 mg/kg BW i.v., Hypnodil (Jansson), 5 mg/kg BW i.v., and atropine (Dispersa), 0.05 mg/kg BW i.v. Intubation was assisted by Succinolin (Amino), 2 mg/kg BW i.v. Then the animals were mechanically ventilated with a 50% nitrous oxide-oxygen mixture at a respiratory rate of 2 l/min and a RMV of 3.5 liters, using a Radcliff machine. Alloferin (Roche), 0.5 mg/kg BW i.v., was given as a relaxant and pethidine (Hoechst) or Nembutal (Abbott), 5 mg/ kg BW i.v., was given for analgesia. The animals were extubated under atropine, 0.05 mg/kg BW i.v., Prostigmin (Roche), 0.25 mg/kg BW i.v., and Novalgin (Hoechst), 50 mg/kg BW i.v. and an equal dose i.m.

33

Table 1. Technique of Anesthesia

	Medication	Route	Dosage
Premedication	Ketalar	i.m.	12.5 mg/kg BW
Induction	Stresnil	i.v.	2 mg/kg BW
	Hypnodil	i.v.	5 mg/kg BW
	Atropine	i.v.	0.05 mg/kg BW
Intubation	Succinolin	i.v.	2 mg/kg BW
Ventilation	Mechanical (Radcliff machine)		21 breaths/min 3.5 l r.m.v.
Inhalation	N_2O/O_2		3:2 to 1:1
Analgesia	Pethidine	i.v.	0.05 mg/kg BW
	Nembutal	i.v.	5 mg/kg BW
Extubation	Atropine	i.v.	0.05 mg/kg BW
	Prostigmin	i.v.	0.25 mg/kg BW
	Novalgin	i.v. and i.m.	each 50 mg/kg BW

2.2 Experimental Design

Division into groups (Tables 2 and 3): The animals were separated into groups on the basis of the variables stated earlier (number of screws and plate length; with or without abutments; mode of placement of abutments; extraoral or combined intra- and extraoral approach; with or without periosteal separation in the area of the alveolar ridge; with or without creation of a skin flap; survival time 3 − 4 months or over 3 years). Five groups were designated:

Group 1 was a control group composed of 7 minipigs (animals 1 − 7) that were not operated on but were maintained under the same conditions as the experimental animals.

Group 2 consisted of 6 minipigs (animals 8 − 13) in which the reconstruction plate with condylar head was inserted through an extraoral approach. The resection was performed 1 − 2 cm proximal to the junction of the chin and horizontal ramus. The reconstruction plates were shortened in animals 8 and 9 and

Table 2. Number of Screws and Mode of Placement of the Abutments Used in the Experiments

Number of screws	Abutment				Number of animals
	None	Trans-mucosal	Trans-alveolar	Trans-osseous	
None	7	−	−	−	7
5− 7 Screws	2	8	−	−	10
9−12 Screws	4	3	10	10	27
Total	13	11	10	10	44

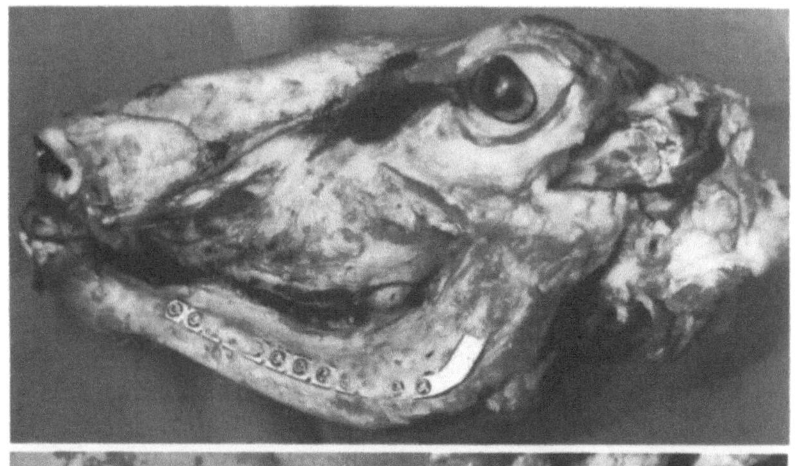
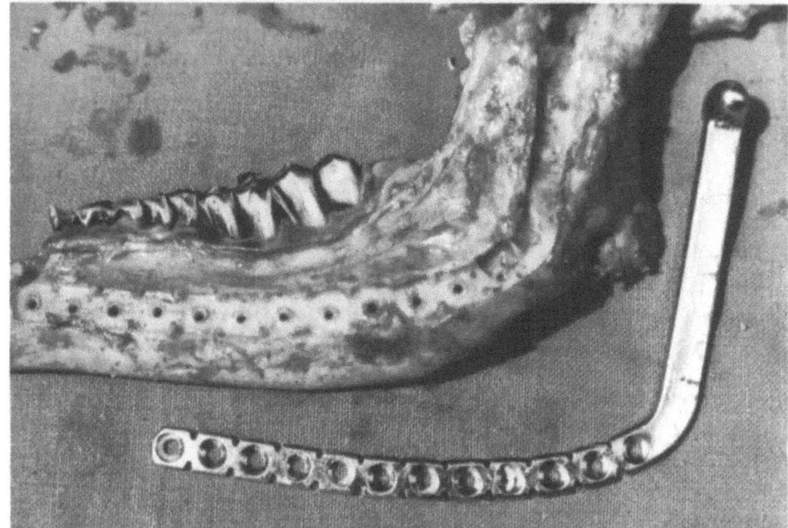

Fig. 48 a, b. Reconstruction plate with condylar head in a sheep 6 months after resection and replacement of the vertical ramus immediately distal to the dental arcade (animal 5). **a** The reconstruction plate is partly covered by bone in the area of the vertical ramus. The bony vertical ramus has been completely regenerated by periosteal bone formation, and the resection site is difficult to identify. **b** Implant bed after removal of the plate. The implant bed and all screw beds are invested by bone

fixed only in the chin area with 5−7 screws. In animals 10−13 the plate was unshortened and extended across the midline to the opposite ramus; it was attached with 9−12 screws.

Group 3 consisted of 11 minipigs (animals 14−24) in which the reconstruction plate with condylar head was implanted through an extraoral approach following a hemimandibulectomy proximal to the chin area. The plate was fixed in the chin area with 5−7 screws in animals 14−21, and across the

Table 3. Overview of the Experimental Design

Group	No. of animals	Animal no.	Resection	Approach	No. of screws	Abutment	Remarks
1	7	1– 7	–	–	–	–	Control animals
2	6	8–13	Transverse, 15 cm	Extraoral	5– 7 9–12	None	Animals 8– 9: ipsilateral anchorage Animals 10–13: anchorage across midline
3	11	14–24	Transverse, 15 cm	Extraoral	5– 7 9–12	Transmucosal	Animals 14–21: ipsilateral anchorage Animals 22–24: anchorage across midline
4	10	25–34	Stepped, 15 cm	Combined intra-/ extraoral	9–12	Transalveolar	Animals 25–29 with Periosteal stripping in area of alveolar Animals 30–34 without ridge
5	10	35–44	Stepped, 13 cm	Extraoral	9–12	Transosseous	Animals 35–39 survival time 3–4 months Animals 40–44 survival time over 3 years

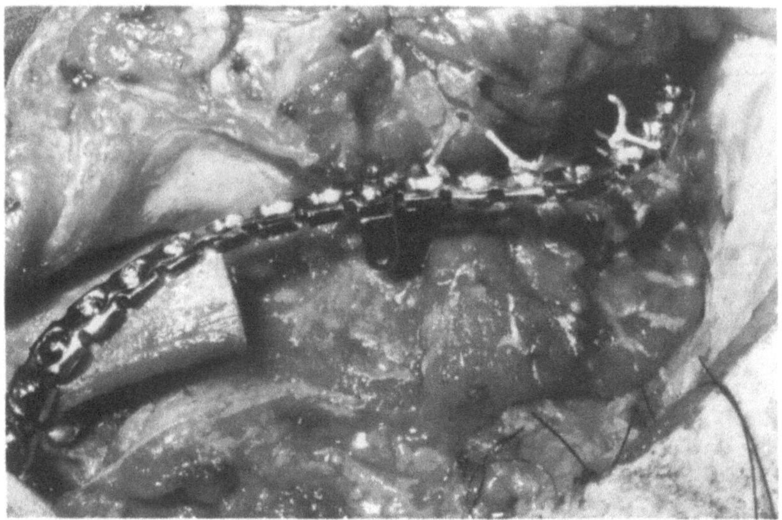

Fig. 49. Operative field in the minipig (animal 16). The left horizontal ramus of the mandible has been resected proximal to the chin, and a reconstruction plate with condylar head has been attached in the ipsilateral chin area with 7 screws. An abutment is fastened to an anchoring element on the plate and projects transmucosally into the oral cavity. The temporalis muscle is fixed to the plate with stay sutures in the area of the mandibular angle

midline with 9−12 screws in animals 22−24. An anchoring element was screwed to the reconstruction plate to permit the attachment of an abutment (Fig. 49) that projected transmucosally into the oral cavity.

Group 4 consisted of 10 animals (animals 25−34) that underwent a preliminary operation in which teeth were extracted through an intraoral route, and the oral mucosa was closed. Then the resection was carried out proximal to the chin area through an extraoral route using a stepped cut. The periosteum was stripped in the area of the alveolar ridge in animals 25−29 and was left intact in animals 30−34. The reconstruction plate with condylar head extended across the midline and was attached with 9−12 screws. A transalveolar abutment was placed through the extraction wound and fastened to an anchoring element on the plate (Fig. 50).

Group 5 consisted of 10 minipigs (animals 35−44) in which the mandibular resection was performed through an extraoral approach with a stepped cut made about 1 cm proximal to the first molar. After removal of the tooth germs contained in the bone, the abutment was inserted transosseously into the oral cavity. The abutment was fastened to the anchoring element of the reconstruction plate with condylar head, which was fixed across the midline with 9−12 screws. Necropsy was performed after the usual 3−4 months in animals 35−39; animals 40−44 were not sacrificed, the intention being to keep them alive for several years to permit a longer-term follow-up.

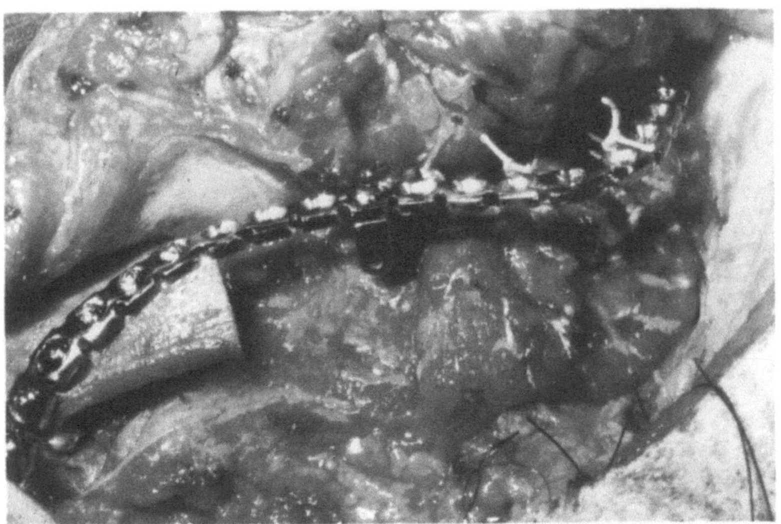

Fig. 50. Site of operation in the minipig (animal no. 25). Stepped resection in the area of the left horizontal ramus. A reconstruction plate with condylar head is fixed through to the opposite side. An abutment is attached to one of the anchoring elements fastened to the plate; after extraction of the tooth it reaches transalveolarly into the oral cavity

2.3 Operating Technique

In the *extraoral approach* for inserting the reconstruction plate with condylar head (Table 4), the skin was washed, shaved, and aseptically prepared. The incision was made from the root of the ear along the vertical ramus and over the mandibular angle to the horizontal ramus and chin, extending across the midline to the horizontal ramus of the opposite side. Soft-tissue trauma was simulated by mobilizing a narrow flap anteriorly, which overlay the plate when the wound was closed (animals 30−39). After division of the platysma and ligature of the facial artery and vein, the facial nerve was identified, isolated, and protected during reflection of the masseter and lateral and medial pterygoid muscles. The neurovascular bundle was ligated in the area of its emergence. The head of the mandible was resected first so that the reconstruction plate with condylar head could be modeled to the mandibular border and around the chin to the opposite side with the aid of bending pliers. Next the hemimandible was resected somewhat proximal to the strongly receding chin, taking care to preserve the gingiva. The resection was performed with a straight or stepped cut (Figs. 49 and 50), depending on the experimental group. The average length of the resected specimen was 13−15 cm. The mucosal borders were doubly sutured from the extraoral field to provide a watertight closure of the widely opened oral cavity. The shortened reconstruction plate with condylar head was fixed in the chin area with 5−7 screws, and the unshortened plate was fixed across the midline with 9−12 screws. All the screw holes were predrilled and

38

Table 4. Operating Technique

	Condylar prosthesis	Reconstruction plate with condylar head
Preparation:	Lat. position, skin shaved and aseptically prepared	
Incision:	2 Incisions: along zygomatic arch, then 1 FW below angle of mandible	1 Incision: from ear along vertical ramus over angle to horizontal ramus and chin, around to horizontal ramus of contralateral side
Dissection:	TM joint, angle of mandible, subperiosteal tunnel between	Exposure of facial nerve, TM joint, and mandible to horizontal ramus of contralateral side
Resection:	Condylar process (4 sheep)	Angle of mandible, sparing inferior alveolar nerve (2 sheep), hemimandibulectomy just proximal to the chin (37 minipigs)
Placement:	Head of prosthesis in glenoid fossa, spike in neck stump, stem on lateral aspect of mandible	Head of prosthesis in glenoid fossa, stem to the chin or to the horizontal ramus of the contralateral side
Fixation:	Screw holes predrilled and tapped; eccentric screws in DC holes, central screws in round holes	Screw holes predrilled and tapped; 5 – 7 or 9 – 12 screws inserted through centers of plate holes
Muscle fixation:		Temporalis, masseter, medial pterygoid muscles fixed to reconstruction plate
Closure:	Masseter, plasysma, skin in layers	

tapped, and the occlusion and condyle–fossa relation were checked continually during attachment of the plate. Insertion of the abutment posts followed, using a transmucosal placement in group 3 (i.e., through the oral mucosa), transalveolar in group 4 (i.e., through the alveolus of an extracted tooth), and transosseous in group 5 (i.e., through the bone in the edentulous region). The abutments screwed into anchoring elements fastened to the roconstruction plate (Figs. 49 and 50).

The masseter and oral floor muscles were approximated to the abutment, anchoring element, and plate with several fixation sutures to eliminate dead space. The tendons and bony insertions of the temporalis, masseter, and pterygoid muscles were attached to the plate with heavy sutures in the area of the mandibular angle in order to seat the head more securely into the glenoid fossa and prevent its dislocation (Fig. 49). This was further aided by passing the masseter-pterygoid sling around the plate and securing it with a suture. Closure was completed in layers at the level of the platysma and skin.

In the *combined intra- and extraoral approach,* a preliminary operation was done in which the teeth were extracted through an intraoral approach. Following mobilization of the mucosa and periosteum, plastic coverage of the alveoli also was undertaken through the intraoral route (Table 4).

2.4 Postoperative Follow-Ups

The various postoperative investigations are listed below:

Postoperative Follow-Ups (first daily, then weekly)
  Body weight
  Temperature and pulse
  Masticatory function
  Sequential dye injections

Gross Postmortem Examination
  Stability of the reconstruction
  Plate seating
  Screw seating
  New bone formation in the resection defect
  New bone formation in the area of the prosthetic anchorage
  Operative scar
  Soft-tissue coverage
  Masticatory muscles
  Tissue surrounding the abutment
  Mucosal coverage
  Implant bed
  Abutment anchorage
  Joint motion
  Joint stability
  Lateral deviation of the mandible

Radiographs
  Axial and lateral

Microscopic Examination of Plate Anchorage, Glenoid Fossa, Abutment Anchorage, Contralateral Temporomandibular Joint
  Undecalcified microtome sections with Goldner stain, $5-7$ µm thick
  Microradiography
  Undecalcified bone sections, $80-100$ µm thick
  Fluorescent microscopy

Table 5. Regimen for Sequential Dye Injections (Polychromic Labeling) in the Minipigs. (After RAHN 1976)

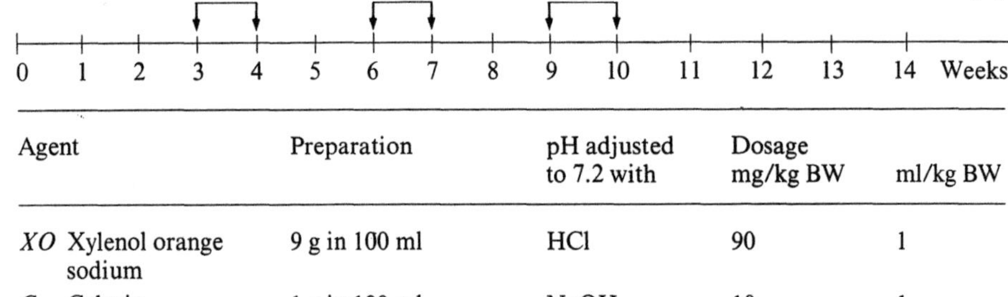

Agent	Preparation	pH adjusted to 7.2 with	Dosage mg/kg BW	ml/kg BW
XO Xylenol orange sodium	9 g in 100 ml	HCl	90	1
C Calcein	1 g in 100 ml	NaOH	10	1
TC Oxytetracycline	Per manufacturer's recommmendations		25	—

Follow-ups in the postoperative period consisted of daily and then weekly measurements of body weight and evaluations of masticatory function. The minipigs continued to receive dry feed. The technique of sequential dye injection ("polychromic labeling") as described by RAHN [84] was used so that the progress of bone remodeling could be evaluated later on. Starting in the 3rd week, the animals received weekly injections of xylenol orange (Siegfried), 90 mg/kg BW, for two weeks, then calcein (Siegfried), 10 mg/kg BW, and finally oxytetracycline, 25 mg/kg BW. The regimen is shown in Table 5.

2.5 Necropsy

Most of the animals were necropsied after 11 – 17 weeks (average 13.3 weeks). First the following parameters were checked and evaluated macroscopically (Figs. 51 – 56):

— stability of the reconstruction,
— plate seating,
— screw seating,
— new bone formation in the resection defect,
— new bone formation in the area of the prosthetic anchorage,
— operative scar,
— soft-tissue coverage,
— masticatory muscles,
— tissue around the abutment,
— mucosal coverage,
— implant bed,
— abutment anchorage,
— joint motion,
— joint stability,
— mandibular deformity.

2.6 Technique of Examination

Necropsy specimens were fixed in precooled 50% alcohol. One week later we obtained an axial radiograph of the specimen and also a lateral radiograph after dividing the mandible anteriorly (Figs. 57 – 59) (see list on p. 40).

The specimens were processed further to obtain undecalcified microtome sections with Goldner stain (5 – 7 μm), microradiographs, and undecalcified bone sections (80 – 100 μm), unstained or spot stained in basic fuchsin, for each mandible from the areas of the plate anchorage, glenoid fossa and abutment (Fig. 60) and from the contralateral temporomandibular joint, following the method of SCHENK [95]. The sequential dye labels were studied by fluorescent microscopy (Figs. 61 – 66; see also p. 40).

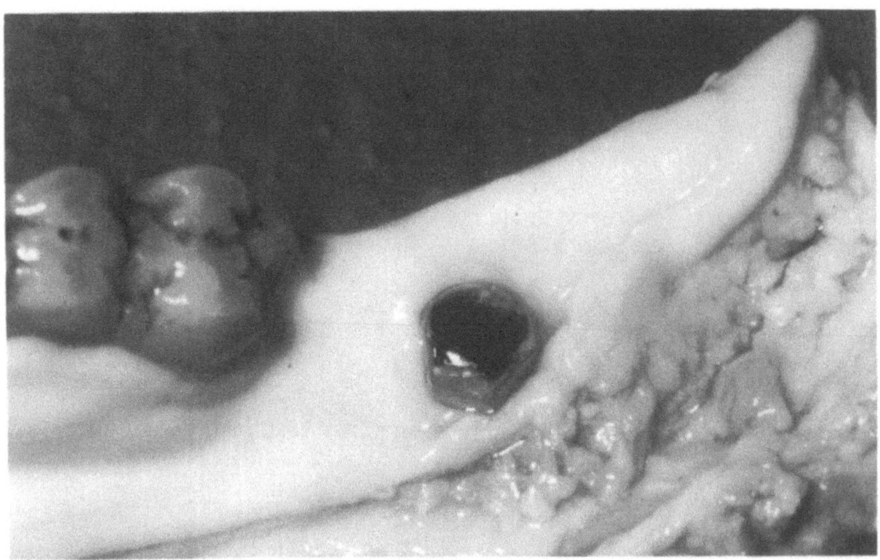

Fig. 51. Transmucosal abutment: necropsy specimen from a minipig 13 weeks after free-end insertion of a reconstruction plate with condylar head attached across the midline and fitted with a transmucosal abutment (animal 22). The mucosa surrounding the abutment is free of irritation

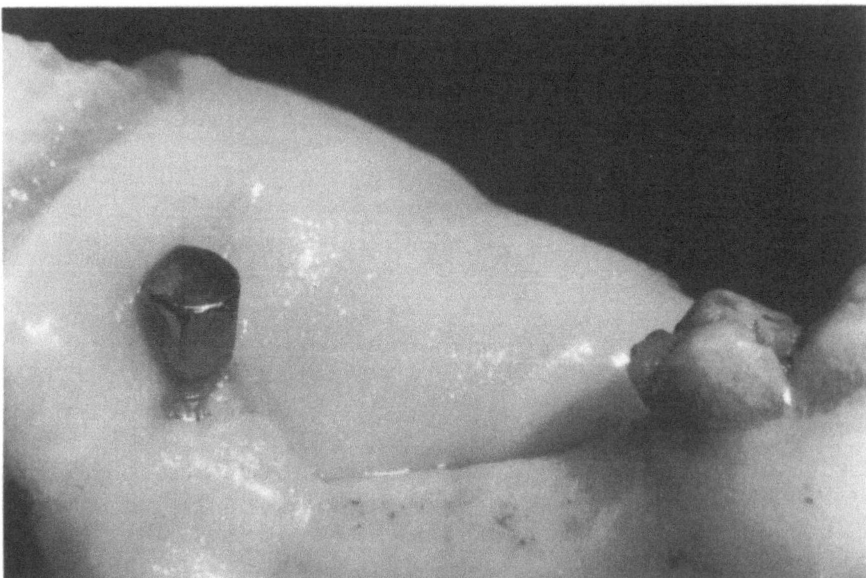

Fig. 52. Transalveolar abutment: necropsy specimen from a minipig 12 weeks after free-end insertion of a reconstruction plate with condylar head attached across the midline and fitted with an abutment placed through the alveolus of an extracted tooth (animal 33). Owing to bone regeneration in the resection defect, the mucosa is somewhat higher distally than mesially in the area of the still healing extraction wound

42

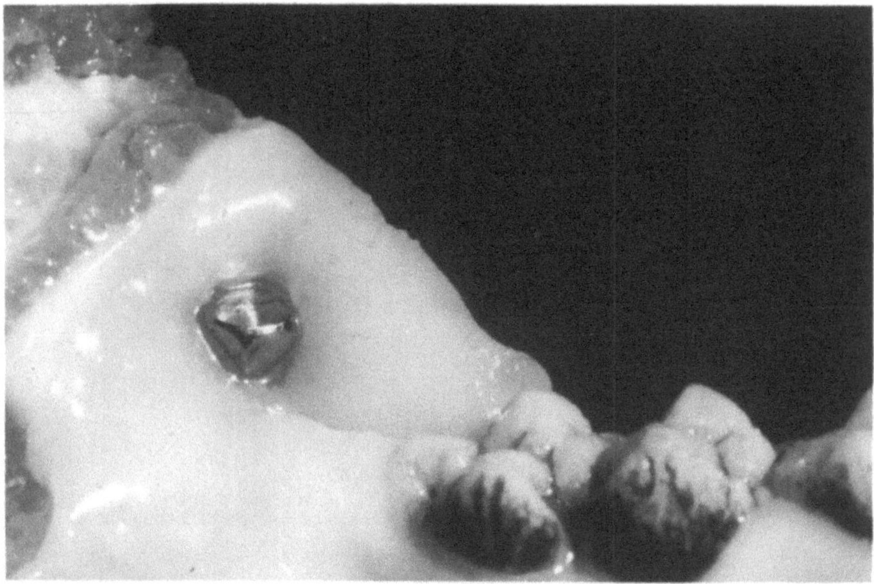

Fig. 53. Transosseous abutment: necropsy specimen from a minipig 11 weeks after free-end insertion of a reconstruction plate with condylar head attached across the midline and fitted with an abutment inserted through the bone (animal 38). The mucosa surrounding the abutment is free of irritation (see also Fig. 59)

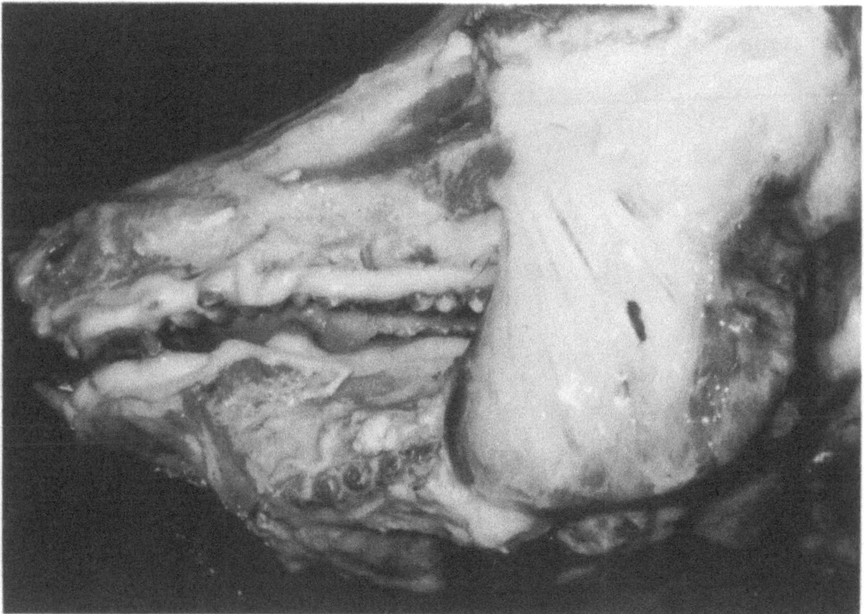

Fig. 54. Postmortem findings in a minipig 15 weeks after operation (animal 12). With functionally stable anchorage of the reconstruction plate with condylar head, the masticatory muscles on the operated side and contralateral side show no signs of atrophy

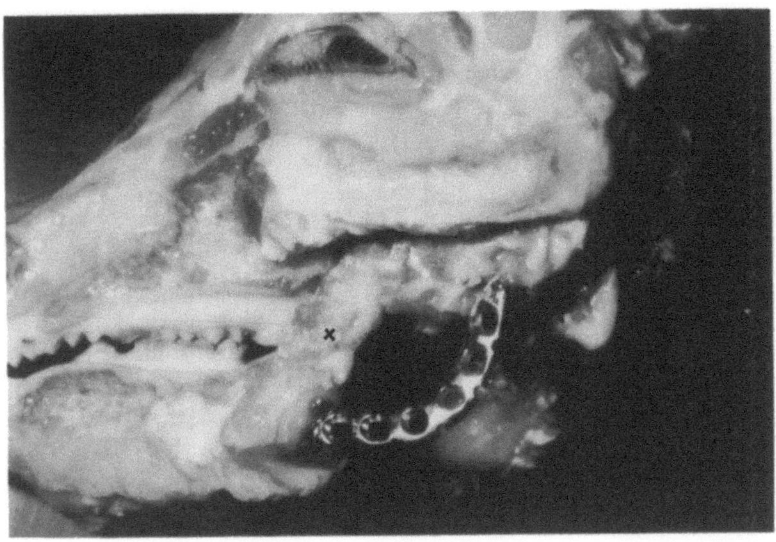

Fig. 55. Postmortem findings in a minipig 13 weeks after free-end insertion of a reconstruction plate with condylar head attached across the midline (animal 27). The regenerated bone (×) completely bridges the defect, indicating functional stability. The new bone occurs mainly along the anterior border of the vertical ramus, a typical configuration for the 4th postoperative month (see also Fig. 58 a)

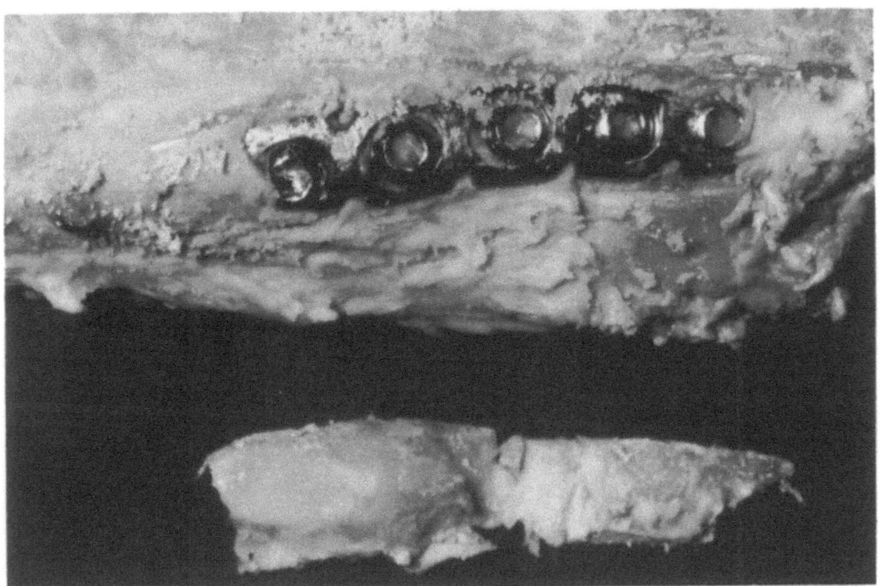

Fig. 56. Necropsy specimen from a minipig 11 weeks after insertion of a reconstruction plate with condylar head (animal 37). The bony shell covering the plate and screw heads has been removed

44

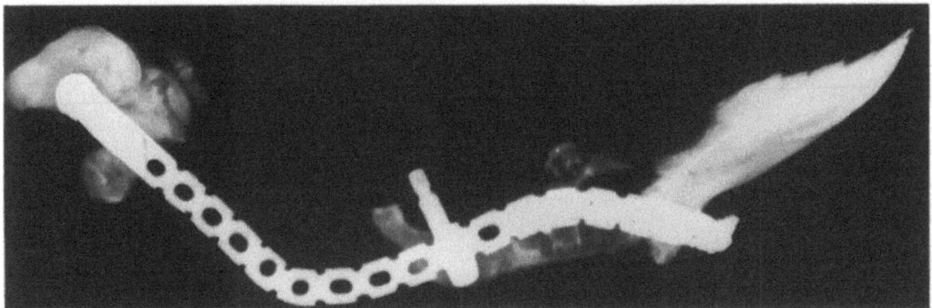

Fig. 57. Lateral roentgenogram of a mandibular specimen divided in the symphyseal area, 16 weeks after a mandibular resection proximal to the chin and insertion of a reconstruction plate with condylar head attached with 7 screws and fitted with a transmucosal abutment (animal 19). Signs of early instability are visible in the chin area, where there is bone resorption under the plate; the screws are not yet loose. Even after 4 months, bone regeneration has not completely bridged the defect, giving further evidence of instability. The newly formed bone in the horizontal ramus extends only to the area of the abutment and its anchorage, which, however, are closely invested by bone. The artificial condyle is also surrounded by a dense area of new bone growth

Assessment of the functional performance of the reconstructed mandible was based on:

1. weight gain (determination of time required to surpass weight at operation),
2. the stability of the reconstruction (assessment of the anchorage of the implant and individual screws),
3. the epithelial margin around the abutment post (determination of the position and status of the tissue surrounding the abutment).

We used a numerical rating scale to evaluate the individual results for each animal as well as the overall results for each group[2], with 1 = good, 2 = satisfactory, 3 = adequate, 4 = poor.

---

2 For weight gain: numerical rating of mean value; for stability and epithelial margin: mean value of individual numerical ratings.

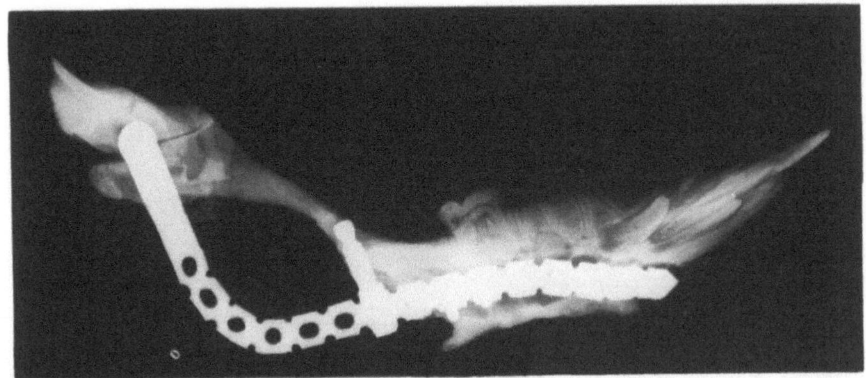

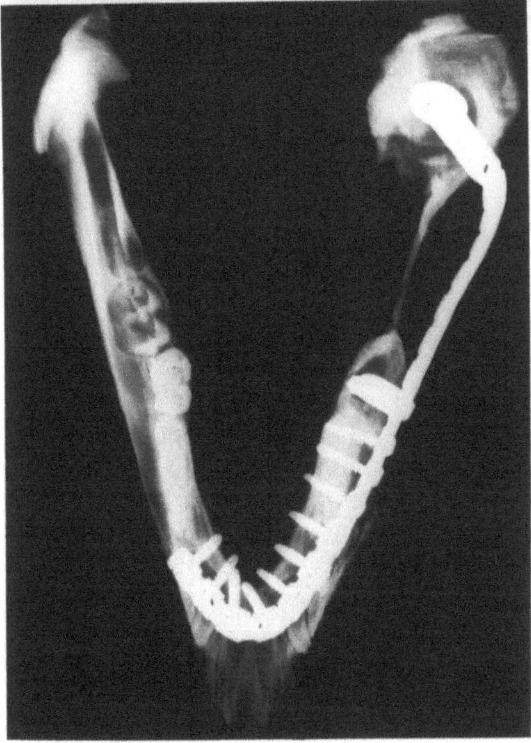

Fig. 58 a, b. Lateral and axial roentgenogram of mandibular specimens (animals 27 and 26, respectively) taken 13 and 12 weeks after mandibular resection in the molar region and insertion of a reconstruction plate with condylar head attached with 12 and 10 screws; both plates were fitted with transalveolar abutments. **a** All screws are stably anchored. Functional stability is evidenced by complete bone regeneration across the defect. The bone invests the abutment not just basally in the area of the anchoring element but also cranially from the original alveolar border (see also Fig. 55). The head of the plate is closely invested by bone. **b** Again, all the screws in this specimen are stably anchored. There is no evidence of bone resorption about the plate and screws. At 12 weeks the defect is spanned by a thin but continuous bony bridge, confirming functional stability; the alveoli around the anchoring element and abutment did not have time to fill completely with bone. The bone of the glenoid fossa is closely apposed to the condylar head

Fig. 60 a, b. Necropsy specimens from a minipig 12 weeks after free-end insertion of a reconstruction plate with condylar head attached across the midline and fitted with a transalveolar abutment (animal 26). **a** Abutment and its anchorage after removal of the plate. **b** Abutment and anchoring element are removed and replaced by a plastic rod so that the specimen will not deform when embedded in methylmethacrylate

46

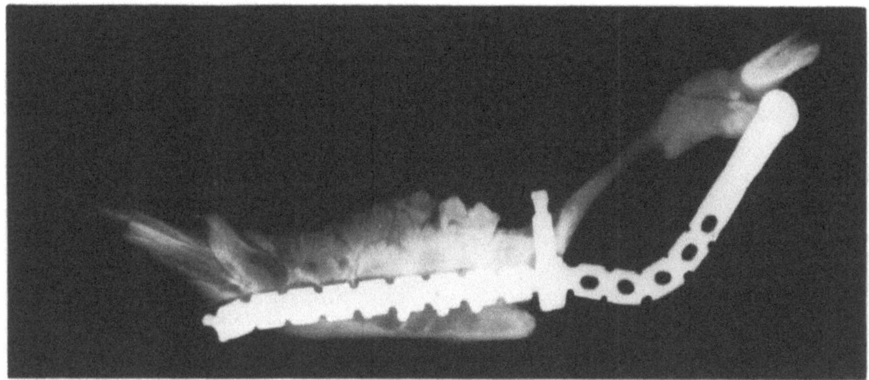

Fig. 59. Lateral roentgenogram of a mandibular specimen divided in the symphyseal area 11 weeks after mandibular resection in the molar region and insertion of a reconstruction plate with condylar head attached with 11 screws and fitted with a transosseous abutment (animal 38). The plate and all screws are radiologically stable, confirming the functional stability of the reconstruction. The defect is completely spanned by regenerated bone, which is very prominent for 11 weeks. The abutment is closely invested by original and new bone (see also Fig. 53). The area of the glenoid fossa is unchanged relative to the unoperated side

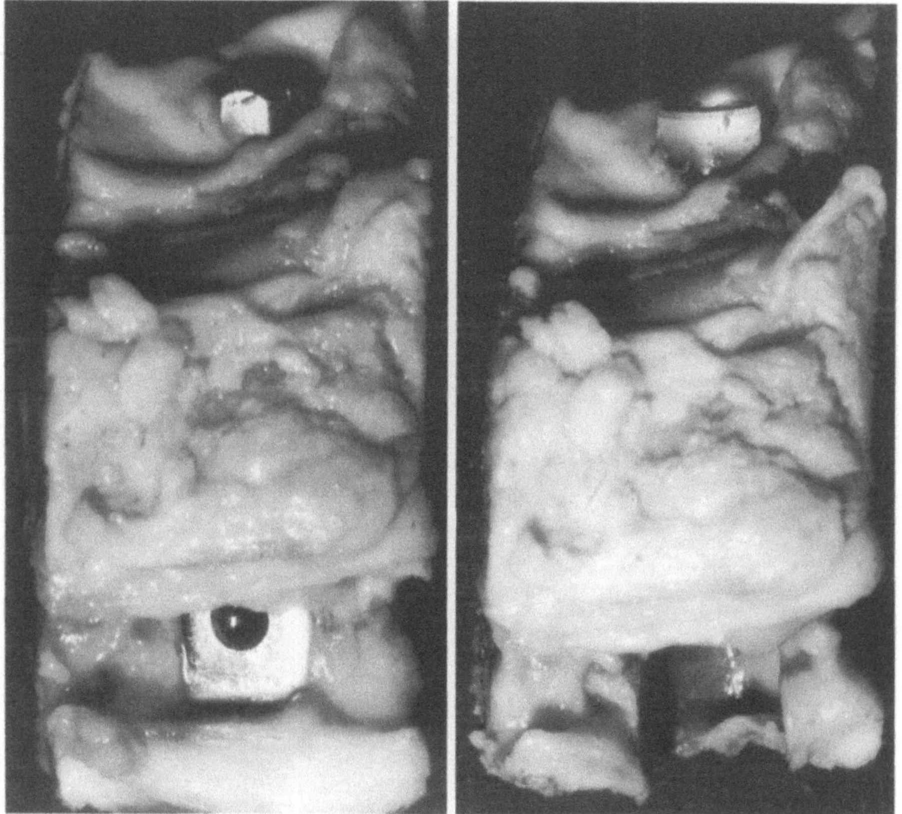

a

b

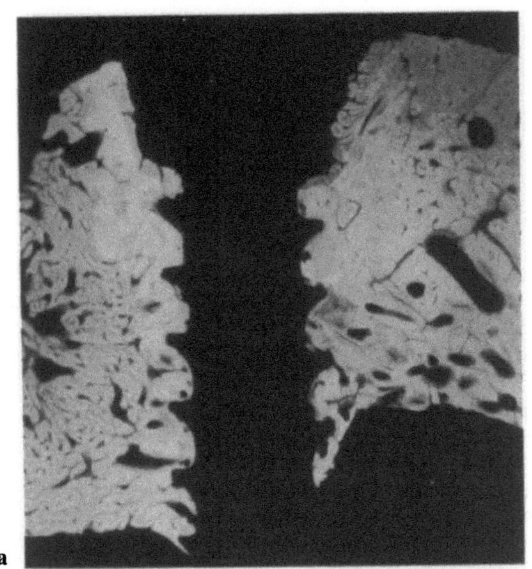

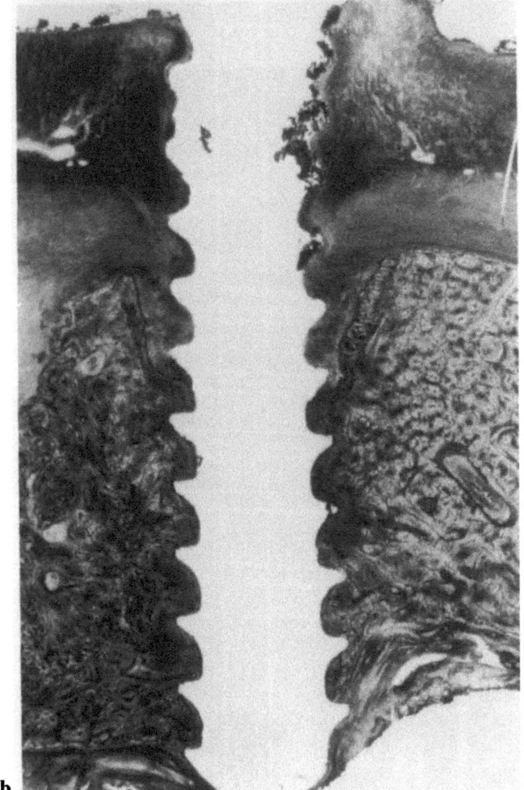

48

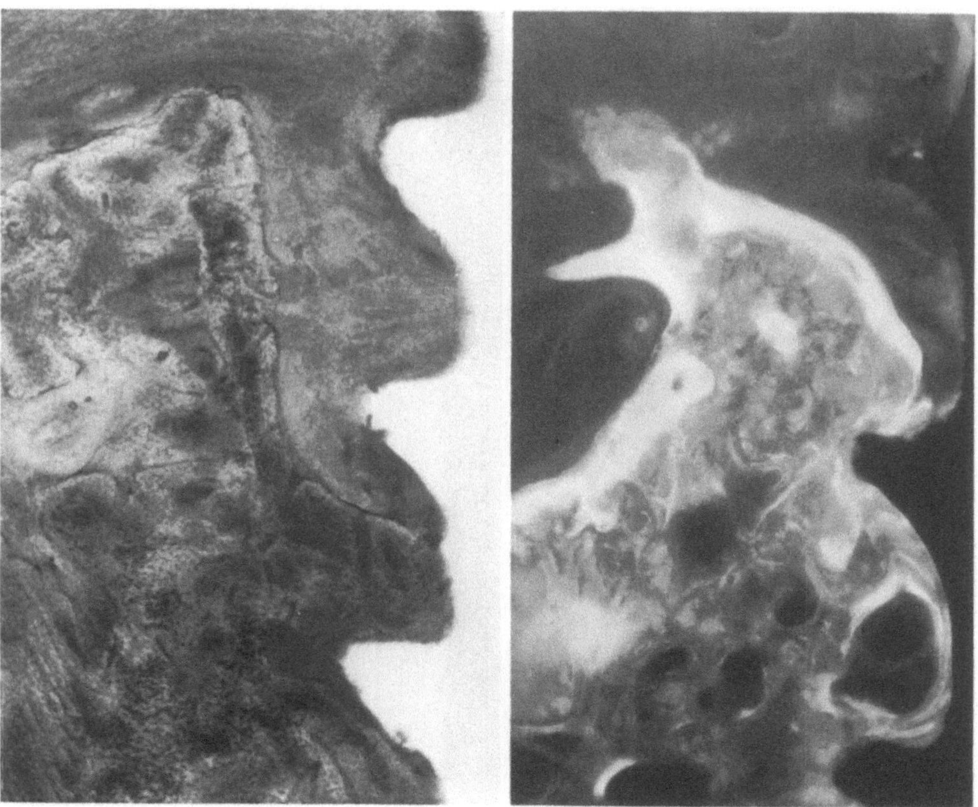

d

Fig. 61 a – d. Plate and screw beds in the horizontal ramus of the minipig 14 weeks after free-end insertion of a reconstruction plate with condylar head attached ipsilaterally with 7 screws (animal 15). There are signs of early instability of the screw anchorage. Note the funnel-like widening of the screw tract about the neck of the screw. Intervening connective tissue is visible around the upper portion of the screw/bone interface, while farther down the bone reaches fully into the interspaces between the threads. Newly formed bone is visible on the ·surface of the osseous threads.

Low- and higher-power views of the screw beds. **a** Microradiograph (9 ×). **b, c** Undecalcified sections spot stained in basic fuchsin (9 × and 36 ×). **d** Fluorescent micrograph of undecalcified section with sequential polychromic labels (45 ×)

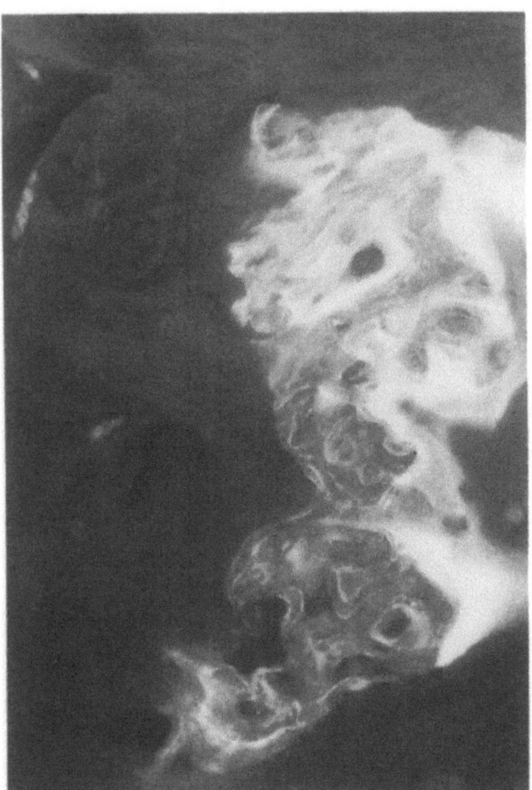

Fig. 62. Plate and screw beds in the horizontal ramus of a minipig 14 weeks after insertion of a reconstruction plate with condylar head attached ipsilaterally with 5 screws (animal 14). Instability is evidenced by a thick connective tissue layer about the plate and screw beds and by obvious signs of bone resorption. Fluorescent micrograph of undecalcified section with sequential polychromic labels (45×)

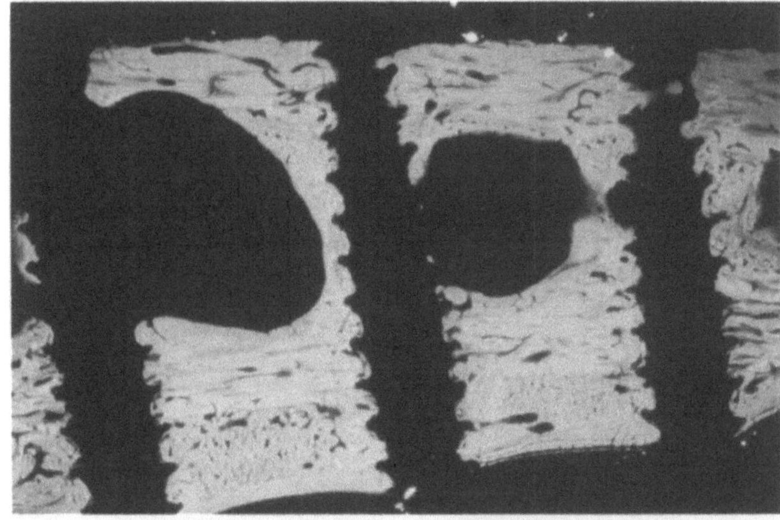

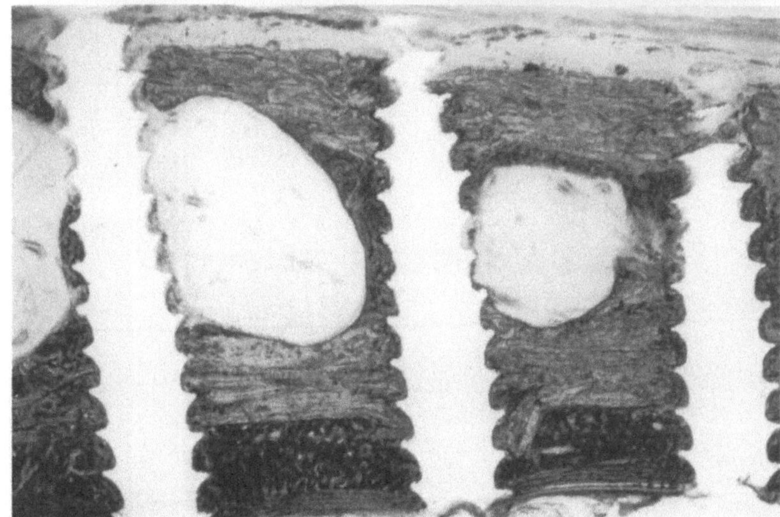

Fig. 63a–e. Plate and screw beds in the horizontal ramus of a minipig 14 weeks after free-end insertion of a reconstruction plate with condylar head attached across the midline (animals 11, 30, and 31). There is evidence of stable screw anchorage in the bone. The bone reaches well into the interspaces between the threads, and there is newly formed bone in the area of the plate bed and on the surface of the bony threads. The sequential injections of xylenol orange, calcein, and oxytetracycline were spaced 3 weeks apart, and each dye was administered twice at weekly intervals, as indicated by the double lines.

Low- and higher-power views of the screw beds. **a, c** Microradiographs (6× and 18×). **b, d** Decalcified sections spot stained in basic fuchsin (6× and 18×). **e** Fluorescent micrograph of undecalcified section with sequential polychromic labeling (45×)

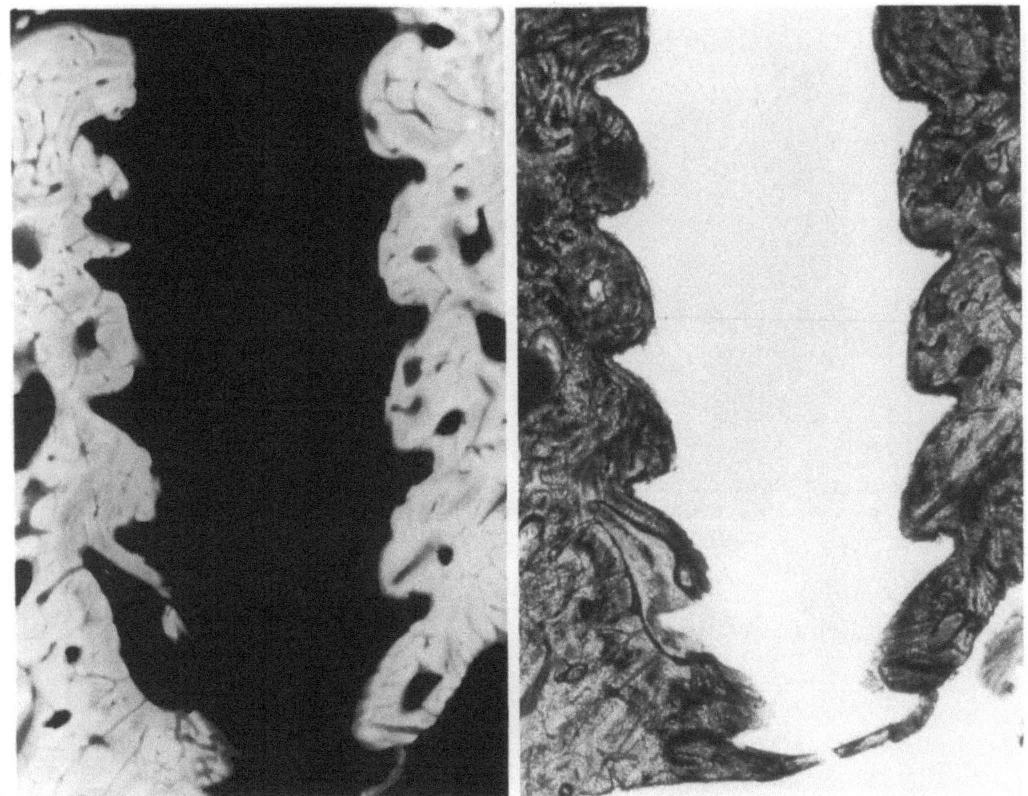

Fig. 63 c, d. (Caption see p. 51)

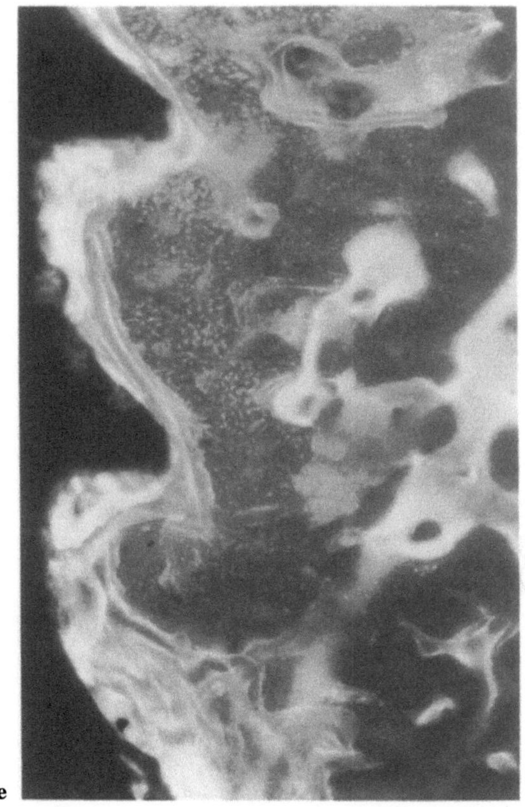

Fig. 63e. (Caption see p. 51)

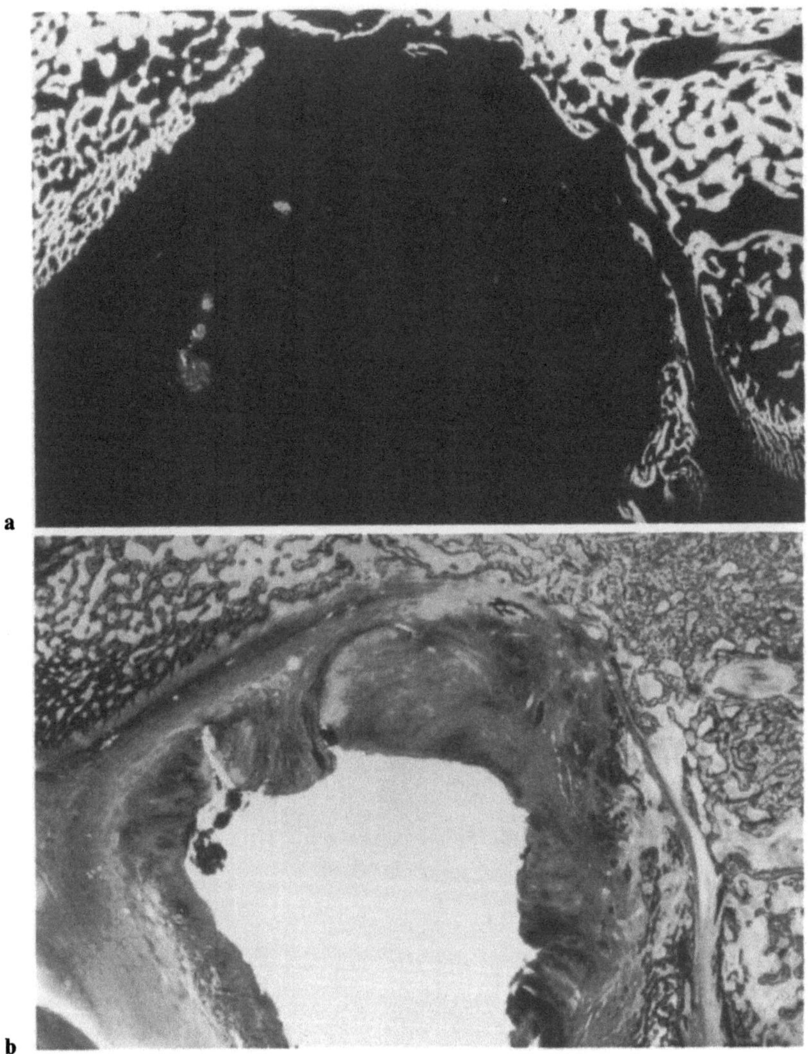

Fig. 64 a, b. Implant bed around the condylar head in a minipig 15 weeks after free-end insertion of a reconstruction plate attached ipsilaterally (animal 9, unstable anchorage). A layer of connective tissue surrounds the condylar head. There is obvious resorption of the underlying bone, and no new bone deposition is apparent below the connective tissue layer. **a** Microradiograph (6×). **b** Undecalcified section, Goldner stain (6×)

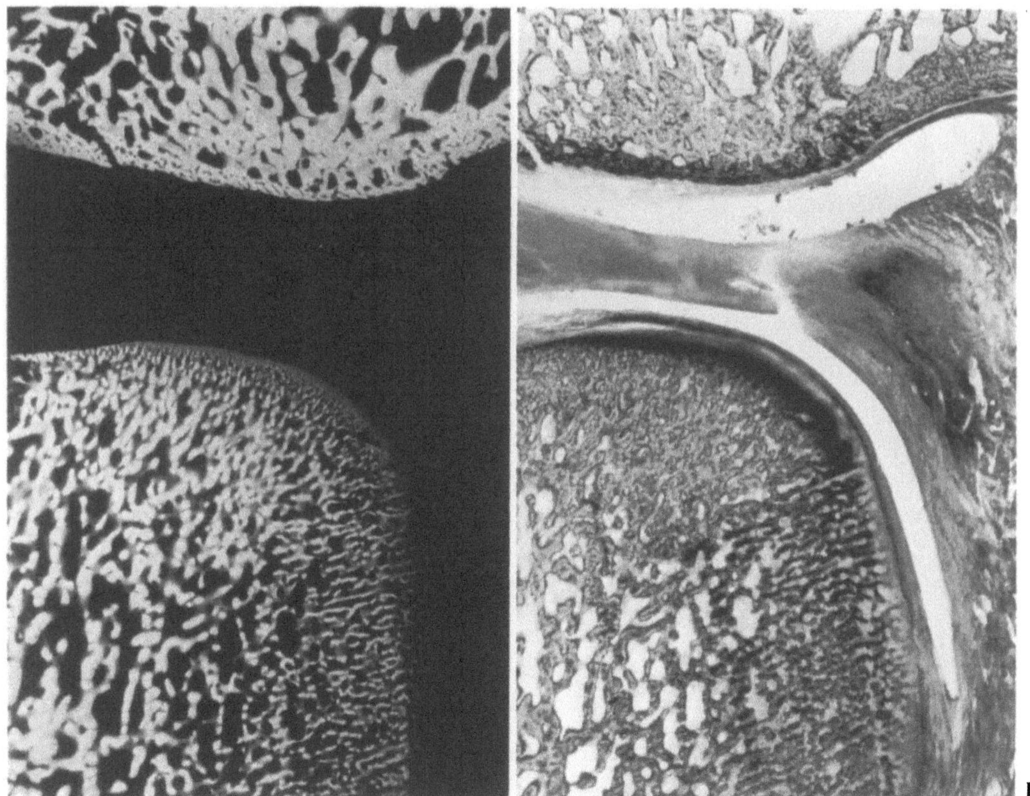

Fig. 65 a, b. Contralateral temporomandibular joint in a minipig 16 weeks after free-end insertion of a reconstruction plate with condylar head attached ipsilaterally. Unoperated side: glenoid fossa, disc, condyle head, insertion of lateral pterygoid muscle. No abnormalities are visible in the configuration or structure of the joint. Growth of the condyle is not yet complete. **a** Microradiograph (6×). **b** Undecalcified section spot stained in basic fuchsin (6×)

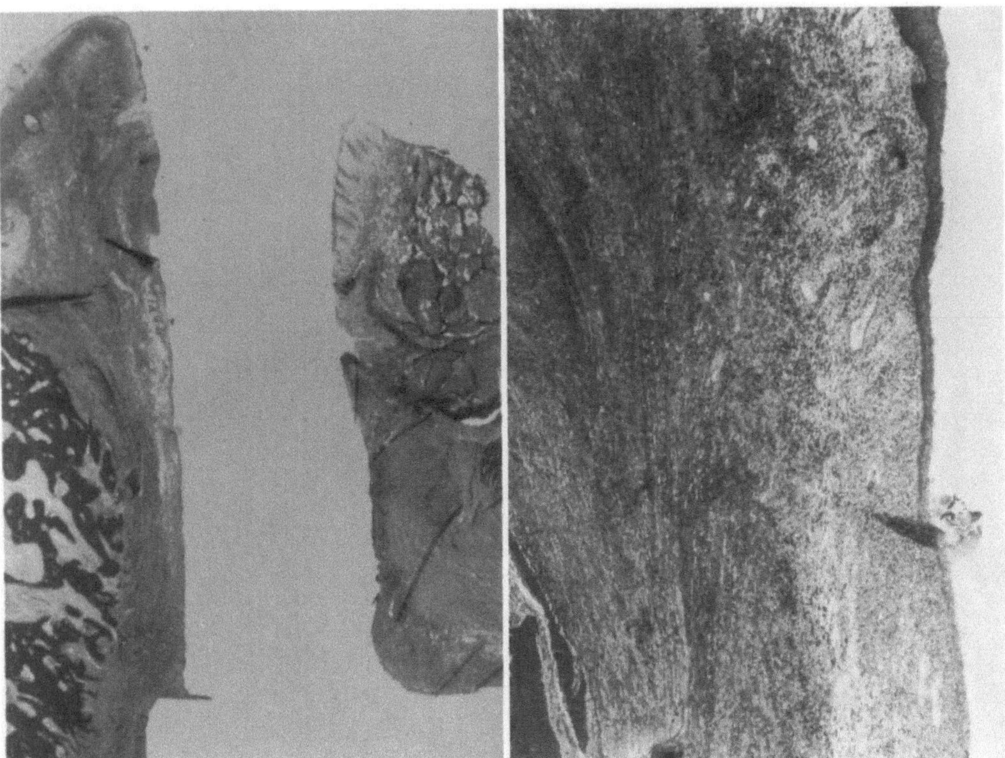

Fig. 66a–d. Tissues about the abutment and anchoring element in minipigs at 16, 13, and 15 weeks (animals 25, 22, 23) after stable anchorage of a reconstruction plate with condylar head, fitted with a transalveolar (animal 25) or transmucosal abutment (animals 22 and 23). The abutment inserted in the area of the resection is surrounded by a connective tissue layer, surrounded in turn by regenerated bone. There is normal apposition of mucosa to the abutment. **a** and **b** show a gradually thinning epithelium invaginating halfway down the transalveolar abutment. In the specimens from the transmucosal abutments (**c** and **d**), the epithelium extends to the abutment neck without downgrowth. There is subperiosteal bone about the abutment neck extending to a point just below the epithelial margin; a thick connective tissue layer is visible farther down, in the direction of the anchoring element. **a** Low-power view of undecalcified section, Goldner stain (6×). **b** Epithelial margin, undecalcified section, Goldner stain (36×). **c** Epithelial margin, undecalcified section, Goldner stain (12×). **d** Epithelial margin, undecalcified section, Goldner stain (24×)

56

c
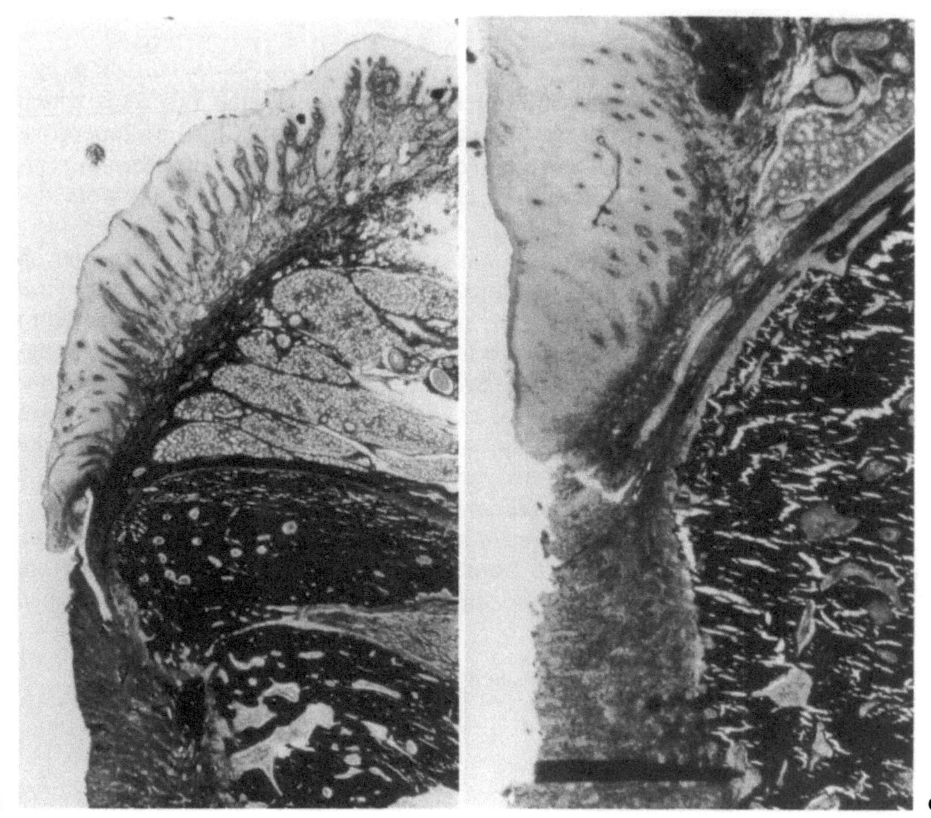
d

Results

Our preliminary experiments showed that bone remodeling processes which critically affect the end result were apparent as early as the third postoperative month. This finding was taken into account in the present experimental regimen. The results of the preliminary experiments (Figs. 47 and 48) were described in an earlier publication [114].

This preliminary observation was confirmed in our experiments on minipigs, for which sequential dye injections from weeks 3 to 10 and a *survival time* of 14 weeks proved favorable. By that time the reconstruction appeared to have reached a state that was more or less definitive in terms of osseous changes and stability. This did not apply to changes about the ipsilateral and contralateral temporomandibular joints, however, especially in animals that were still growing. Because the long-term success of an articular prosthesis in the clinical setting requires at least 10 years' follow-up, 5 animals from group 5 were kept alive for longer-term observation.

Systemic complications not directly related to the mandibular reconstruction occurred in 6 animals. Animal 6 from the control group and animal 36 from group 5 died with *Hemophilus* infection; a similar, nonfatal infection developed

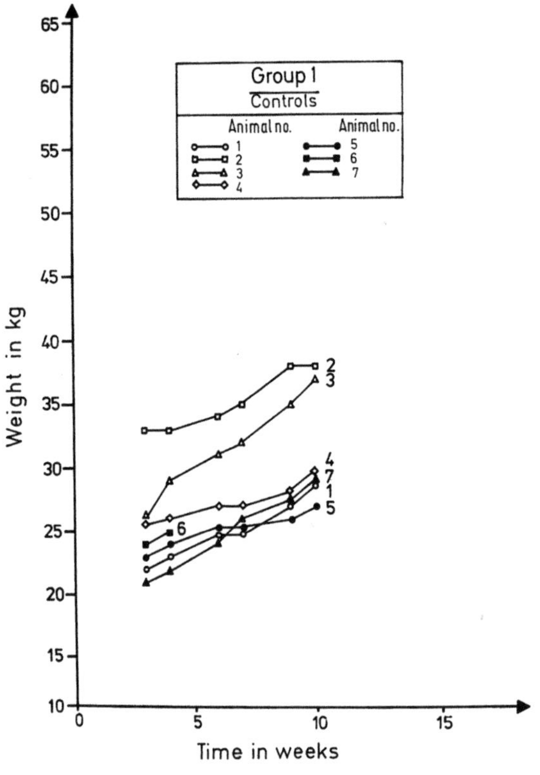

Fig. 67. Weight gain in control animals 1−7 (group 1). Animal 6 died from a *Hemophilus* infection. The remaining animals exhibited steady weight gains

in animal 39 from group 5, and animal 13 from group 2 contracted a pneumonic infection. *Complications not related to the experiment* developed in 2 animals. Animals 24 and 32 from groups 3 and 4 sustained a mandibular fracture caused by a mishap during injection of the dye. This led in animal 24 to a loosening of the plate anchorage and subsequent infection, so that the displaced reconstruction plate finally was attached only to the fractured, devitalized fragment. This animal lost a total of 3 kg. In animal 32 the undisplaced fracture occurred outside the area of the plate anchorage.

Only a few days after surgery these animals exhibited a normal *masticatory function* and ate their customary dry feed. In no case was intermaxillary fixation applied.

Weight gain showed a temporary decline in the operated animals, contrasting with the continuous rise in the untreated controls (Figs. 67−71). It took an average of 3−9.5 weeks, depending on the group, for the body weight to surpass the weight at operation (Table 6). The greatest differences were associated with different modes of plate fixation (5−7 screws placed in the chin area vs. 9−12 screws placed across the midline). The presence or absence of an abutment, the mode of placement of the abutment, and the choice of surgical approach (extraoral or combined intra- and extraoral) caused only minor discrepancies. When we rate the time required to surpass weight at operation on a numerical scale[3] (Tables 6 and 7), we obtain the following results for the different variables (the number of animals to which the result pertains is given in parentheses):

Control animals	1 (n = 6)
Operated animals	2 (n = 28)
Fixation with 5−7 screws	4 (n = 10)
Fixation with 9−12 screws	2 (n = 18)
Without abutment	2 (n = 5)
With abutment	2 (n = 23)
Transmucosal abutment	3 (n = 10)
Transalveolar abutment	2 (n = 10)
with periosteal stripping	2 (n = 5)
without periosteal stripping	1 (n = 5)
Transosseous abutment	1 (n = 3)
Extraoral approach	2 (n = 8)
Combined intra-/extraoral approach	2 (n = 10)

The attainment of *functional stability* was a major problem whose solution lay in adopting the correct insertion technique. Functional stability was assessed at weekly follow-ups on the basis of radiographs (Figs. 57−59) and at necropsy by macroscopic (Figs. 51−56, 60) and microscopic examination (Figs. 61−66).

---

3 Time required to surpass weight at operation:
   1 = 0−3 weeks   3 = 7−9 weeks
   2 = 4−6 weeks   4 = more than 10 weeks

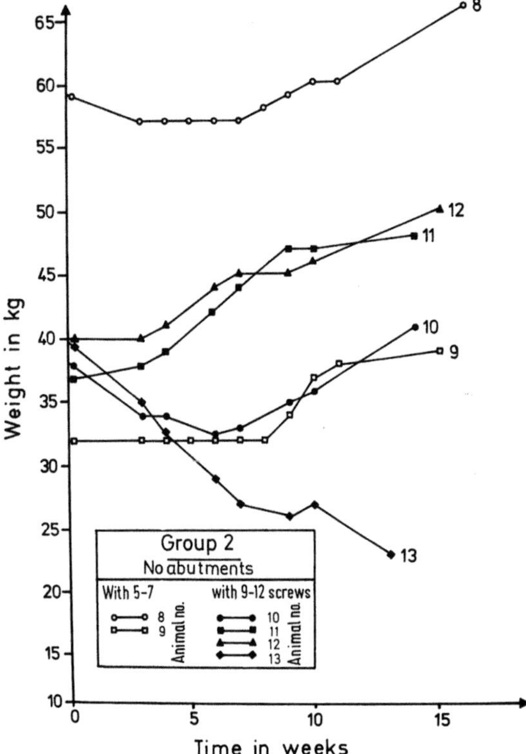

Fig. 68. Weight gain in animals 8−13 (group 2) (transverse resection, extent of resection 15 cm, extraoral approach, no abutments, fixation with 5−7 screws in animals 8 and 9, with 9−12 screws in animals 10−13). Animal 13 developed a pneumonic infection and lost weight. Animals 8−10 initially lost weight after surgery and required about 10 weeks to regain their operative weights. Animals 11 and 12 began gaining weight only 3 weeks after surgery, but at a somewhat slower rate than the controls

The results showed that fixation of the implant with 5−7 screws in the ipsilateral chin area was inadequate to achieve a functionally stable anchorage. Plate loosening occurred within a few weeks under masticatory loads. Unstable seating of the plate and screws was apparent at necropsy (Figs. 57, 61, 62). The plate loosening manifested itself in local infections and changes in the soft tissues and operative scar involving fistula formation and dehiscence, especially anteriorly. These lesions did not resolve, in contrast to the superficial necrosis caused by deficient blood flow, like that occurring in the skin flap mobilized to simulate soft-tissue injury. Periosteal bone regeneration in the region of the defect failed to produce a continuous bony bridge (Fig. 57). In some cases incipient instability caused an increased periosteal bone reaction in the area of the plate anchorage. The masticatory muscles showed signs of moderate atrophy.

When the plate was anchored across the midline with 9−12 screws, gross examination disclosed a stable implant anchorage with solid seating of the plate and screws (Figs. 54−56, 58, 59), and histologic examination consistently showed the bone to be in intimate contact with the screws (Fig. 63). The skin and mucosa remained intact. Superficial necrosis associated with circulatory compromise in the anterior soft-tissue flap resolved quickly. The operative scar was free of irritation, and at necropsy we were unable to tell which side had

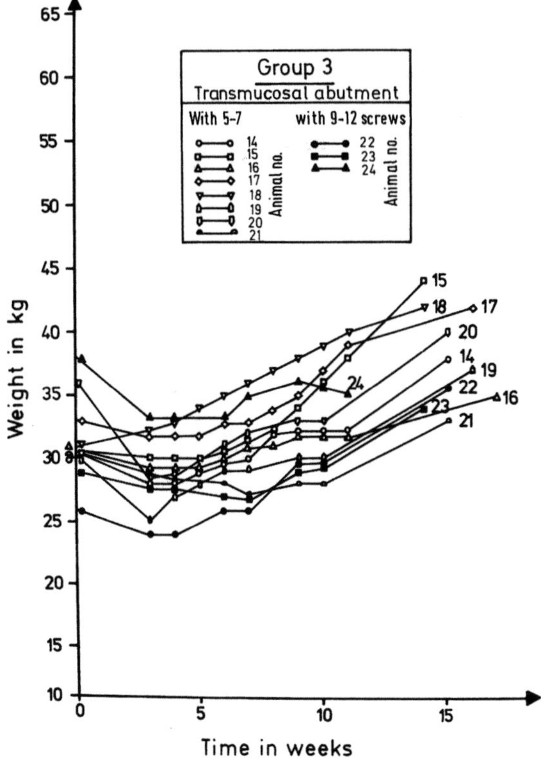

Fig. 69. Weight gain in animals 14−24 (group 3) (transverse resection, extent of resection 15 cm, extraoral approach, transmucosal abutment, fixation with 5−7 screws in animals 14−21, 9−12 screws in animals 22−24). Animal 24 sustained a mandibular fracture in a fall during the dye injection and lost weight after a period of initial gain. The remaining animals exhibited a steady weight gain after an initial postoperative loss

been operated by external inspection alone. The masticatory muscles appeared well developed (Fig. 54).

Bone regeneration arising from the periosteum bridged the surgical defect from the mandibular stump below the anterior border of the masseter muscle to the remnant of the articular process and temporalis tendon (Figs. 50, 55, 58, 59). The sequential dye injections showed that the regeneration progressed rapidly at first, then at an increasingly slower pace. New bone formation finally led to complete osseous bridging of the defect in all cases where a functionally stable plate anchorage was obtained.

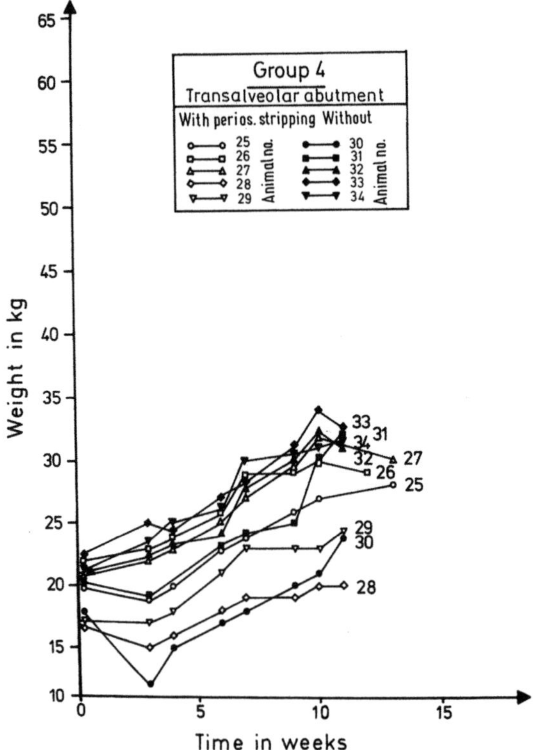

Fig. 70. Weight gain in animals 25–34 (group 4) (stepped resection, extent of resection 15 cm, combined intra-/extraoral approach, transalveolar abutment, fixation with 9–12 screws). Animal 32 fell during the dye injection, sustaining a mandibular fracture which subsequently healed. Except for animal 30, the curves showed little or no postoperative weight loss. The animals quickly reassumed a normal pattern of weight gain

When functional stability was rated on a numerical scale[4] (Tables 6 and 7), it was found to correlate markedly with the mode of plate fixation but showed no dependence on other variables:

Fixation with 5–7 screws	3	(n = 10)
Fixation with 9–12 screws	1	(n = 23)
Without abutment	2	(n = 5)
With abutment	1.4	(n = 28)
Transmucosal abutment	2.1	(n = 10)
Transalveolar abutment	1	(n = 10)
With periosteal separation	1	(n = 5)
Without periosteal separation	1	(n = 5)
Transosseous abutment	1	(n = 8)
Extraoral approach	1.1	(n = 13)
Combined intra- and extraoral approach	1	(n = 10)

---

4 1 = Implant and all screws solid
   2 = Implant solid; a few screws show signs of loosening
   3 = Implant loose but undisplaced
   4 = Implant loose and displaced

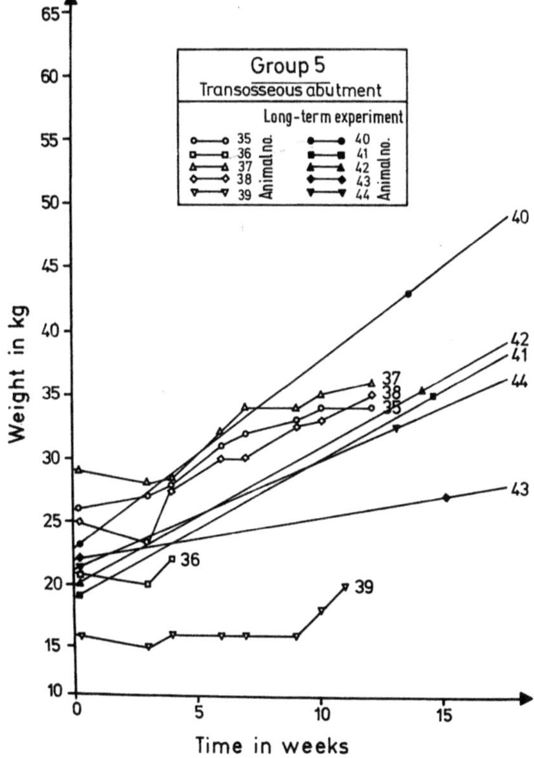

Fig. 71. Weight gain in animals 35–44 (group 5) (stepped resection, extent of resection 13 cm, extraoral approach, transosseous abutment, fixation with 9–12 screws). Animal 36 died from a *Hemophilus* infection. The postoperative weight gain was slight and of very short duration. Weight determinations in the 5 animals in the long-term experiment were made at longer intervals

Both macroscopic (Figs. 51–53) and microscopic examination (Fig. 66) showed that the condition of the tissue about the abutment, especially the quality of the *epithelial seal,* was influenced greatly by the stability of the plate anchorage. Instability led to pocket formation down to the abutment anchorage (animals 15, 17–21) and in one case (animal 14) allowed epithelial downgrowth around the plate itself.

With a stable plate anchorage, both the transmucosal abutments (animals 22 and 23, Figs. 51, 66c, d) and the transosseous abutments (animals 35, 37–39, Fig. 53) developed an epithelial seal that was free of irritation and pockets. With one exception (animal 43), the animals with transosseous abutments that were not necropsied (animals 40–44) likewise showed an irritation-free epithelial margin when examined clinically under general anesthesia. In the case of the transalveolar abutments, good results were mixed with several cases of slight epithelial invagination with pocketing. On the one hand this was due to the formation of sequestra (animals 28, 29) in cases where, following a stepped resection and periosteal stripping, the alveolar wall was connected to the mandibular stump mesially by only a narrow bridge of bone (animals 25–29). Another cause was dehiscence in the area of the dental extraction wound, whereupon the alveolus filled with granulation tissue and underwent secondary

Table 6. Individual Results of the Numerical Ratings

Group	1		2		3		4		5	
Number of animals	7		6		11		10		10	
Systemic complications	1[a]		1[b]		1[c]		1[c]		2[a, d]	
Results	1:	1−X−X	8:	4−3−X	14:	3−3−4	25:	2−1−2	35:	1−1−1
	2:	1−X−X	9:	3−3−X	15:	3−2−3	26:	1−1−1	36[a]:	X−X−X
Animal no.:	3:	1−X−X			16:	3−2−2	27:	1−1−1	37:	2−1−1
weight gain-stability-	4:	1−X−X	10:	4−2−X	17:	3−2−3	28:	2−1−2	38:	2−1−1
epithelial margin	5:	1−X−X	11:	1−1−X	18:	1−2−3	29:	2−1−2	39[d]:	4−1−1
	6[a]:	X−X−X	12:	2−1−X	19:	4−2−3				
	7:	1−X−X	13[b]:	4−3−X	20:	4−3−3	30:	3−1−1	40:	X−1−1
					21:	4−3−3	31:	2−1−1	41:	X−1−1
							32[c]:	1−1−1	42:	X−1−1
					22:	3−1−1	33:	1−1−1	43:	X−1−2
					23:	4−1−1	34:	1−1−2	44:	X−1−1
					24[c]:	4−4−4				

Explanation of numerical rating scales (X = no rating, no result)

Weight gain:

1 0−3 ⎱ Time in weeks
2 4−6 ⎰ required to
3 7−9 ⎰ surpass weight
4 10 ⎰ at operation

Stability:

1 Implant and all screws solid
2 Implant solid; a few screws show signs of loosening
3 Implant loose and undisplaced
4 Implant loose and displaced

Epithelial margin:

1 Irritation-free, tight epithelial seal at the level of the abutment
2 Pocket formation by epithelial invagination; epithelial seal at the level of the abutment
3 Epithelial invagination to the abutment anchorage
4 Epithelial invagination to the implant with exposure of the abutment anchorage

Example:

18: 1−2−3 means that animal 18 surpassed its weight at operation within 3 weeks; the implant was solidly seated, with a few screws showing evidence of loosening; there was epithelial downgrowth to the abutment anchorage.

[a] Died from *Hemophilus* infection; [b] Pneumonic infection; [c] Mandibular fracture from fall during dye injection; [d] Contracted *Hemophilus* infection

Table 7. Numerical Ratings of the Group Results

Material			Variables		Results			
Group	Animal no.	Number of animals	Number of screws	Abut-ment	Weight gain	Sta-bility	Epithe-lial margin	Overall result
1	1– 7 without 6	6	–	–	1	X	X	1
2	8–13 without 13	5 2 3	5– 7 9–12	None	4 2	3 1.3	X X	3.5 1.7 2.6
3	14–24 without 24	10 8 2	5– 7 9–12	Trans-mucosal	3	2.4 1	3 1	2.8 1.7 2.2
4	25–34 without 32	10 5 5	9–12	Trans-alveolar	2[a] 1[b]	1[a] 1[b]	1.6[a] 1.2[b]	1.5[a] 1.1[b] 1.8
5	35–44 without 36 and 39	8 3 5	9–12	Trans-osseous	1 X	1 1	1 1.2	1 1.1 1

See Table 6 for explanation of rating scale.
[a] With periosteal stripping
[b] Without periosteal stripping

epithelialization (animals 25, 29, 34, Fig. 66a, b). Sequestra did not form in cases where the periosteum of the alveolar walls was left intact (animals 30–34).

A numerical rating of the quality of the epithelial margin[5] around the abutment posts (Tables 6 and 7) yielded the following results:

Fixation with 5–7 screws	3 (n = 8)
Fixation with 9–12 screws	1.3 (n = 20)
Transmucosal abutment	1 (n = 2)
Transalveolar abutment	1.4 (n = 10)
With periosteal stripping	1.6 (n = 5)
Without periosteal stripping	1.2 (n = 5)
Transosseous abutment	1.1 (n = 8)
Extraoral approach	1.1 (n = 10)
Combined intra- and extraoral approach	1.4 (n = 10)

Because the experimental results were affected so critically by the *mode of fixation* of the reconstruction plate with condylar head, we felt justified in disregarding the 10 animals with 5- to 7-screw, ipsilateral fixation when evaluating the remaining variables, and we focused our attention on the 23 animals in which the plate had been anchored across the midline with 9–12 screws.

The numerical rating of the mode of fixation (Tables 6 and 7) yielded the following results:

---

5 1 = Irritation-free, epithelial seal at the level of the abutment
   2 = Pocket formation by epithelial invagination; epithelial seal at the level of the abutment
   3 = Epithelial invagination to the abutment anchorage
   4 = Epithelial invagination to the implant with exposure of the abutment anchorage

	5−7 screws	9−12 screws
Weight gain	4 (n = 10)	2 (n = 18)
Stability	3 (n = 10)	1 (n = 23)
Epithelial margin	3 (n = 8)	1,3 (n = 20)

The *abutment* caused few problems. The attachment of the abutment to the reconstruction plate (Fig. 44) showed satisfactory stability in all cases. Abrasions on the teeth mesial to the resection site and on the maxillary antagonists of the abutment (with a chipped-off cusp in animal 28) confirmed masticatory function on the resected side. Apparently the risk of infection was not increased by the open connection from the oral cavity along the abutment post and anchorage to the plate (animals 14−44). In any case, infection did not develop in any of the animals that had a functionally stable plate anchorage (animals 22−44). We observed no instance of ascending infection to the temporomandibular joint. Infection was a problem only when instability was present and occurred in the area of loose screws, in pockets about the abutments, and in the area of bony sequestra. Rating the results on a numerical scale for reconstructions with and without abutments (Tables 6 and 7) in the 23 animals that had 9- to 12-screw anchorage of the plate across the midline yielded the following results:

	Without abutment (n = 3)	With abutment (n = 20)
Weight gain	2	1.9 (u = 15)
Stability	1.3	1

Results varied with the *mode of placement of the abutments,* i.e., with their transosseous vs. transalveolar or transmucosal insertion. The alveolar process, which was mobilized during the stepped resection of the base of the mandible, showed a marked dependence on the blood flow through the periosteum. Stripping of the periosteum retarded postoperative weight gain and impaired the epithelial seal around the abutment as a result of sequestration. On the other hand, failure to mobilize the mucosal periosteum led to some difficulties in sealing the alveolus, so that secondary healing of the dental extraction wound impaired the epithelial seal at the abutment (Fig. 52). Transmucosal insertion of the abutment, while favorable in terms of stability and epithelial seal, appeared to compromise masticatory function on the resected side due to a lack of osseous support for the gingiva. This was reflected in a significant delay of weight gain. Cases stabilized with 9−12 screws were rated as follows for different modes of placement of the abutments (Tables 6 and 7):

Abutment:	Transmucosal (n = 2)	Transalveolar (n = 10)			Transosseous (n = 8)
Periosteal stripping		With (n = 5)	Mean	Without (n = 5)	
Weight gain	3	2	1.5	1	1 (n = 3)
Stability	1	1	1	1	1
Epithelial margin	1	1.6	1.4	1.2	1.1

The *operative approach* in the animal experiments − purely extraoral vs. combined intra-/extraoral − had no significant effect. Our numerical rating (Tables 6 and 7) yielded the following results:

	Extraoral approach	Combined intra-/ extraoral approach (n = 10)
Weight gain	2.4 (n = 8)	1.6
Stability	1.1 (n = 13)	1
Epithelial margin	1.1 (n = 10)	1.4

The occurrence of *decubitus ulcers and dehiscence* over the plate showed a dependence on the experimentally restricted blood supply to the anterior soft-tissue flap, on the contouring of the plate at the mandibular angle, and on the stability of the reconstruction. With a well-fitted and stably anchored plate, only one case of decubitus occurred. Superficial necrosis in the area of the mobilized flap resolved without sequelae. The presence of instability led to persistent dehiscence with fistula formation.

Articular function remained intact in all operated temporomandibular joints, with no instances of dislocation or ankylosis. Passive joint motion was found to be unrestricted at necropsy. Grossly and histologically the artificial condylar head was invested by a connective tissue layer of variable thickness, surrounded in turn by zones of bone formation and resorption (Figs. 57−59, 64).

The *contralateral temporomandibular joint* showed no qualitative changes relative to controls (Fig. 65). A quantitative assessment proved difficult because of the imprecisely defined sectional plane. Morphometry during the growth period showed approximately 0.05 mm/week of periosteal bone deposition around the glenoid fossa, and about 1 mm/week of chondral bone formation in the area of the condylar head, with extreme values of 0−1.6 mm. Statistical evaluation of the quantitative data would not have been valid because of inability to define the sectional plane. In the still-growing animals, growth on the control side was on the order of 1 cm during the 4-month period. Examination for mandibular asymmetry showed no deviation that would hamper occlusion in functionally stable reconstructions. Significant mandibular deformity was noted only in association with severe implant loosening.

Table 8. Stages in the Development of the New Implants

	Intermediate stages			Final stage
Dimensions	3.2 · 12 mm		2.5 · 10 mm	2.7 · 7.8 mm	2.7 · 7.8 mm
Deformability	Without notches	Without notches	V-shaped notches 1.5 mm wide, 1 mm deep	V-shaped notches 1 mm wide, 1 mm deep	U-shaped notches 2 mm wide, 1.5 mm deep
Hole spacing	15 mm	8 mm, staggered	8 mm	8 mm	8 mm
Hole shape	Standard DC holes	Round holes		Round holes	Bidirectional DC holes
Location of notches			Horizontal limb to within 10 mm of mandibular angle	Horizontal limb to the mandibular angle	To midportion of the vertical limb
Shape of prosthetic head			Spherical	Bispherical transverse oval 9 mm · 13.5 mm	Bispherical transverse oval 9 mm · 13.5 mm
Neck			10 mm	10 mm	11 mm
Baseplate			12 · 13.5 mm	12 · 13.5 mm	7 · 11 mm
Spike			Angular	6 mm long, 3 mm diam.	4 mm long, 2.3 mm diam.
Stem/neck offset			5 mm	5 mm	4.2 mm
Bending pliers			Combination pliers for bending on the flat and edgewise, two bending irons	Two pliers for edgewise bending and for twisting	Two pliers for edgewise bending and twisting, pliers for bending on the flat
Plate hole accommodates 3.5-mm screw with 2.7 head or lag screw	No		No	No	Yes

The experimental studies affirm the *universal adaptability* of the implants. We were able to adapt the reconstruction plates very readily to all the mandibular contours that were encountered. In 1 case (of a total of 44) the plate fractured while being contoured to the mandible.

We had no difficulty with the postmortem *removal* of the reconstruction plate with condylar head, the anchoring elements, or the abutments themselves. All of the screws came out of the bone intact.

As new discoveries were made during the course of the experiments, the implants underwent continual *modifications* (Table 8). These involved improving the dimensions and bendability of the plates; spacing the plate holes closer together; developing "bidirectional" DC holes; increasing deformability past the mandibular angle; improving the shape of the condylar head, spike, and cervical baseplate of the condylar prosthesis; improving the design of the bending pliers; manufacturing bending templates to aid contouring of the plates; modifying the plate holes to accommodate screws with a 2.7 head and 3.5-mm thread; and designing special spherical-head nuts and a drill guide for attaching the reconstruction plate on the lingual aspect (Fig. 72).

Discussion

To date no animal studies have been published on the reconstruction of large mandibular defects followed by the immediate resumption of masticatory function. In earlier animal studies [133] it was not possible to undertake a mandibular reconstruction without intermaxillary fixation. The resulting compromise of food intake made it necessary to place the animal on a special diet. Reports have been published on the anchorage of preprosthetic abutments in experimental animals with mandibular defects [13–15]. In these studies the abutments were placed only after the incorporation of a bone graft that had been previously prepared to receive the abutment.

1 Discussion of the Method

Because the main problem was to develop reconstruction plates that applied the principles of functionally stable fixation [2, 3, 31, 69–71, 81, 82, 96–98, 137] to the unique mechanical conditions of the mandible [100, 101, 104, 105, 107; 129], our animal experiments were designed to parallel clinical experience and clinical requirements (see lists on p. 19), taking into account the critical assessment of preexisting methods (see p. 17) in the literature [9, 12, 19, 41, 45, 50, 140]. We did not conduct in vitro loading tests to supplement the material tests by the manufacturer, because we feel that load stability depends chiefly on the behavior of the material in response to individual contouring, on its corrosion resistance in the physiologic milieu, on proper anchorage to the mandibular stump, and on the reaction of the material to the unique mechanical conditions in the lower jaw. In vitro testing could not have yielded a clinically meaningful

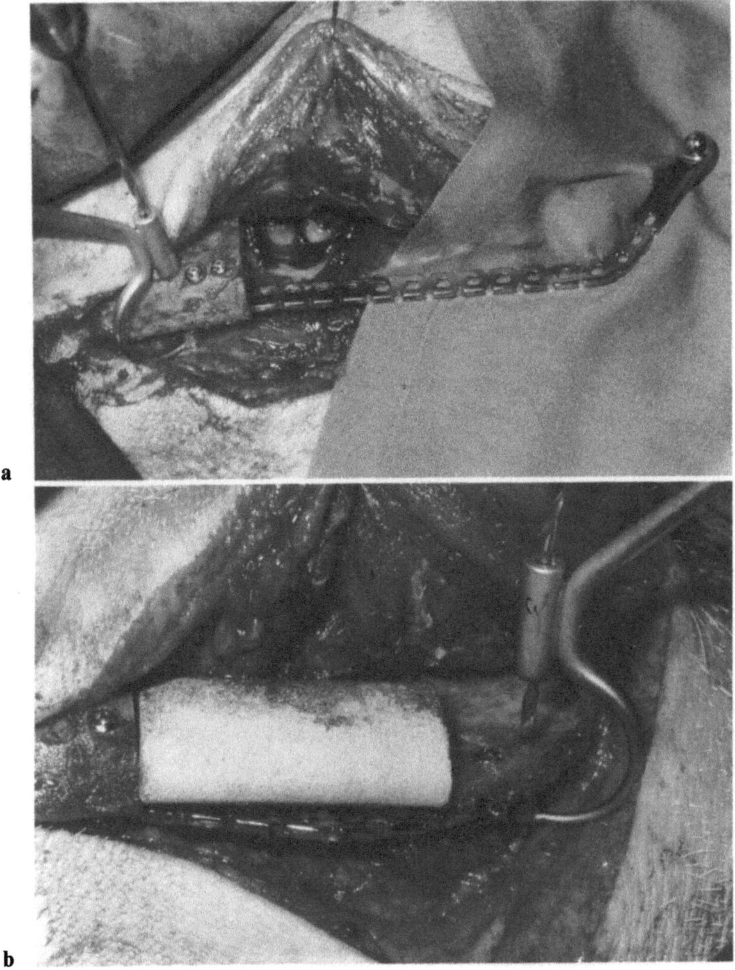

Fig. 72 a, b. Operative field in the minipig. **a** Attachment of a reconstruction plate with condylar head to the lingual aspect of the mandible after hemimandibulectomy in the molar region. The openings of the double DC holes face lingually during adaptation of the plate. A special drill guide is used to drill holes 2.7 mm in diameter (gliding holes). The screw heads appose to the buccal aspect of the bone, while spherical-head nuts seat into the double DC holes of the plate; as stop mechanism keeps them from rotating when the screws are tightened. Attaching the plate lingually lessens the danger of decubitus ulceration of the soft tissues, especially in the area of the mandibular angle. **b** A ceramic implant has been wedged between the mandibular stumps following attachment of the plate on the lingual side. A drill guide is used to drill a 2.7-mm gliding hole at the correct site on the proximal stump through one hole of the reconstruction plate. The holes closest to the defect are already occupied by screws and lingual nuts with rotation stops

result without disproportionately great expense. The concurrent clinical testing of the implants prior to the completion of experimental studies departs from the usual sequence of in vitro testing – animal experimentation – clinical trials. But we felt that such an approach was justified by previous positive experience with ASIF plates in the functionally stable bridging of defects in the extremities, and also by our own experience in the compression plating of mandibular fractures.

We chose the minipig as our experimental animal. Compared with the essentially grinding mastication of the sheep and shearing mastication of the dog, we found that the masticatory action, loading, shape, and bone structure of the mandible in the minipig most closely approximated those in human beings.

The resection of 13–15 cm corresponds to the extent of the mandibular defect that might be expected to result from tumor resection in human patients. In contrast to animal studies involving resections of only 1–1.9 cm [34, 85, 89], a defect of this size permits meaningful testing of the functional stability of a mandibular reconstruction. The essential challenge of mandibular reconstructions is to accomplish the functionally stable bridging of extensive mandibular defects that exceed 12 cm.

The objective criteria that we used to evaluate the success of the reconstruction were weight gain, the periosteal reaction in the area of the resection, and the epithelial investment of the abutment. In preliminary experiments on sheep [114] we found that the animals began to regain weight a short time after operation in cases where a functionally stable implant anchorage was achieved. To evaluate the result of a mandibular reconstruction quantitatively on the basis of body weight curves, it is necessary to use animals that are still gaining weight and to avoid special dietary measures.

Our second criterion of success involved a phenomenon observed in previous animal experiments [133] – a periosteal bone reaction in the presence of functional stability that stimulates bone to regenerate across the resection defect and bridge it completely. Animal studies [133] as well as clinical observations [4, 38, 48, 51, 53] demonstrate that this can occur only if the periosteum is left intact in the area of the resection.

The fact that one-third of the experimental animals were still growing and that the bone resection spared the periosteum could distort the experimental result. But the conditions selected do not compromise the value of the experiment. Growth of the control side relative to the reconstructed side in the immature animals had no deleterious effects during the period of the experiment. The periosteal bone reaction did not affect stability at any time during the experimental period. The conditions during the observation phase, in which a weight-bearing osseous bridge had not yet formed, corresponded well to clinical conditions in adult patients, even when it has been necessary to include the periosteum in the resection. Here bone grafting is manditory if the defect is to become consolidated. The revascularization and functional remodeling of such a graft relies on absolute immobilization by functionally stable fixation between the mandibular stumps; and this immobility in our animal models was manifested most strikingly by periosteal regeneration of the resected bone.

In rating the success of the operation, then, the time required to surpass weight at operation, the bridging of the defect by periosteal new bone formation, and the nature of the epithelial investment of the abutment under the conditions stated offer a sensitive measure of the functional soundness of the reconstructed jaw.

Clinically, a tumor-related mandibular defect often necessitates a course of radiation therapy. The present experimental studies are intentionally limited, at least for the time being, to general principles of mandibular reconstruction. But they also apply in principle to reconstructions after radiotherapy. Indeed, adequate stability can be a very high priority conern in irradiated tissue. Clinical experience teaches that the use or nonuse of radiation after resective therapy does not have a critical bearing on the problem at hand — the functionally stable bridging of an osseous defect with an implant. The most serious problems in the treatment of irradiated tumor patients relate to the healing of bone grafts and the healing of irradiated soft tissues, which frequently have to be replaced with healthy soft tissues by plastic surgery. Animal studies are currently underway to investigate the behavior of irradiated soft tissue over an alloplastic mandibular prosthesis without transfering healthy soft tissue into the area of the defect.

The observation of bone deposition on the implant material raises the question of removability. In our view the removability of implants is of greater concern than the type of bone deposition that occurs, which has already been investigated [120, 121]. The smooth surface structure of the polished ASIF stainless steel enables the implant to be removed without the bonding problems associated with ingrowth into the voids of a titanium sprayed surface.

2 Discussion of Results

The shape of the weight curve is an important criterion of success. To understand this aspect of our experiments more clearly, it should be noted that minipigs 6−8 months of age and weighing 30−35 kg are fully mature skeletally, although their body weight continues to increase. Of the animals that underwent surgery and necropsy, 12 were less than 6 months old at operation, 10 were from 6 to 8 months old, and 10 were older than 8 months. Thus, more than one-third of the animals were still growing during the observation phase, and almost two-thirds were fully mature; thus the experiments were done on fully grown animals as well as animals that were still in their growth period.

The weight curves generally show a more or less prolonged arrest of weight gain in the operated animals compared with the nonoperated controls. Once weight gain has resumed, the weights of the operated animals differ little from one another and from the controls. The different body weights at operation indicate that the weight of the animals starts at different points on the growth curve. As a result, there is no point in making a quantitative comparison of the rise in the weight curves, while the duration of the arrest of weight gain appears to be largely independent of the different ages of the animals. Hence, our main interest from a quantitative standpoint was to establish the time required for the animals to surpass their initial body weight at operation. This period varied significantly from one group to the next and especially in relation to the controls.

Another important criterion of success is the quality of osseous regeneration. Continuous bridging of the mandibular defect by periosteal bone regeneration [4, 9, 38, 51, 53] confirmed functional stability in all the implants that had been attached to the mandible with 9–12 screws. This is an important result, because in the animals whose implants were fixed with only 5–7 screws, osseous regeneration failed to bridge the defect completely.

Additional evaluations of functional stability were based on analysis of the implant bed, screw anchorage, and the reactions of the ipsilateral and contralateral joints, made visible by sequential dye injections [84] and documented by microscopic, radiographic, and histologic studies. The articular changes, marked on the operated side by the formation of a connective tissue layer of variable thickness around the head of the implant with areas of bone formation and resorption, and on the contralateral side by lack of change relative to the controls, remained slight, although changes in the young animals tended to be more rapid and pronounced than in the older animals.

The occurrence of dehiscence anteriorly or at the mandibular angle was, with one exception, referrable to functional instability of the implant anchorage, as with other fixation systems [12, 42, 60, 92]. The single case of dehiscence at the mandibular angle in the presence of a stably bridged defect was caused by overcontouring of the plate, and there was associated decubitus ulceration of the soft tissues stretched over the plate. (Similar lesions have been described in connection with the use of oversize implants [12, 52, 135].) This emphasizes the importance of undercontouring the plate [59] or of fixing the plate to the lingual side when soft-tissue coverage is questionable [109]. A relationship between stability and soft-tissue coverage was also noted in the cases where a narrow anterior skin flap had been mobilized. This area of diminished viability was created to simulate soft-tissue damage resulting from radiation or extensive mobilization. Areas of superficial necrosis as well as more extensive apical flap necrosis with plate exposure resolved completely within a few weeks in the implants fixed with 9–12 screws; soft-tissue dehiscences associated with instability persisted.

Much controversy surrounds the use of surgical approaches that create a communication with the oral cavity. In our animal experiments, there was no evidence that the combined intra-/extraoral approach increased the risk of infection compared with the purely extraoral approach. The same observation has been made by other authors [27–29, 49, 68, 72, 73–78, 91], but on the basis of clinical experience obtained under more favorable conditions of oral hygiene.

Regarding the removability of the implants, we must draw a basic distinction between implants with a continuous surface to which the bone becomes more or less closely apposed, depending of surface properties, and implants with a metallic meshlike structure that becomes permeated by bone ingrowth and thus can be removed only with sacrifice of bony substance. We believe that the ability to remove an implant without inflicting bone damage greater than that already produced by the screw holes is a desirable prerequisite for clinical use. Certainly the range of clinical applications is limited for an implant that is not removable, or whose removal necessitates an extensive osteotomy [12, 45, 85]. There is no question as to the superiority of removable implants as long as they provide adequate stability.

The key to problem-free removal is screw fixation. Only this method offers the advantages of simple, atraumatic fixation plus the excellent primary stability afforded by axial compression. Anchoring elements in the form of a metallic mesh, which becomes bonded to the bone through ingrowth, have a relatively poor primary stability and are difficult to remove.

Surface structure is an important determinant of the ease or difficulty of implant removal. Clinical experience with rigid internal fixation has shown that with titanium screws, which have a rougher surface than the smoothly polished ASIF implant steel, the bonding forces caused by the intimate contact between implant and bone can cause the screw head to break off when removal is attempted. An even stronger bonding effect occurs with materials that have a porous surface.

The attachment of abutments directly to the reconstruction plate following mandibular reconstruction without bone grafting led to satisfying results in our animal experiments. Epithelial downgrowth around the abutment, anchoring element, and plate did not occur in functionally stable reconstructions, and infection was not a problem despite the open communication with the oral cavity. We found that the quality of the epithelial margin depended on the quality of the tissue seal in the area of the abutment. Thus, adhesion of the tissue to the abutment would be desirable around the intraoral base of the post, and a titanium sprayed surface would be advantageous.

The abutment posts projected freely into the oral cavity and did not support a denture. Loading was predominantly vertical or transverse, depending on the nature and intensity of the contact between the posts and their antagonists, which began to elongate a short time after operation. Some of the opposing teeth showed prominent abrasions from occlusal contact with the abutments, indicating that some of the abutments were subjected to extreme loads. However, the experiments did not simulate the actual load conditions that would be associated with the presence of a denture.

In compiling and analyzing the results of the experiments, we made use of numerical scales to rate the individual results (see Table 6). We defined criteria of success for the main clinical parameters (weight gain, stability, epithelial margin) and rated them on a scale from 1 (good) to 4 (poor). Our experimental design was such that it did not permit a statistical analysis of the results of the weight curves. On the one hand, the number of experimental animals is insufficient given the multivariable nature of the problem. On the other, our animal studies were not just for the purpose of evaluating existing hypotheses; a more important goal was to develop new ideas for improved implant designs and surgical techniques suitable for clinical application. Thus the present experimental program extended over a prolonged period as the results of earlier studies laid the necessary groundwork for the experiments that followed. A more randomized approach would be needed to make a meaningful statistical

74

evaluation. A "time effect" was at work, which enabled animals operated near the end of the series to profit from improvements in the reconstruction plates (compare, for example, Fig. 48 with Figs. 41 and 55, or Fig. 47 with Fig. 39) and also from learning by the experimenters.

3 Clinical Significance

The selected experimental design, using an animal with a human-like jaw morphology and masticatory loads, enables us to draw clinical inferences, especially with regard to the development and improvement of the implants and the refinement of operating technique (Table 9). The present experiments show that an extensive bone defect in the mandible of 5- to 12-month-old minipigs not receiving intermaxillary fixation or special dietary measures is an excellent model for investigating the functional stability of reconstructive procedures. There is obvious clinical significance in the modifications made in the shape, dimensions, and ease of handling of the implants and the development of associated instruments and an improved technique. It must be emphasized that the results depend mainly on the functional stability that is obtained. The selection of animals that were still gaining weight (fully mature or still growing) and the conservation of the periosteum while resecting the bone are a reflection of the fact that our primary emphasis was on the investigation of functional stability, which was visibly manifested by early postoperative weight gain and periosteal bone regeneration across the surgical defect. The minimum number of plate screws established in our animal studies cannot be applied directly to human patients, although it is clear that the rate of complications increases when an insufficient number of screws are used.

Also of clinical importance are the nature and extent of plate deformation. When a plate is adapted to the jaw prior to resection, there is a danger that it will impinge too severely on overlying soft tissues, resulting in pressure lesions. This can be avoided either by undercontouring the plate when adapting it to the mandible or by attaching it on the lingual side. Excessive deformation of the plate, either by initial modeling or subsequent functional loading, carries a danger of plate fracture. An angle of 15° between adjacent holes is considered to be the maximum tolerance limit for plate bending. Knowledge that the plate will break on greater deformation can be utilized to shorten a too-long implant by repeatedly bending it back and forth at the desired site by an amount exceeding the safe limit. A simpler alternative is to use the special plate-cutting pliers. Our animal experiments showed that the plates possessed adequate fracture resistance under functional loading despite previous deformation, thus confirming another important prerequisite for clinical use, especially in the case of the reconstruction plate with condylar head. We also found that the bending pliers could be used to center the head in the glenoid fossa even after the reconstruction plate had been definitively attached.

It is clinically significant that the reconstructions using a purely extraoral approach fared no better than those using a combined intra-/extraoral approach. In the latter cases, care was taken to effect a secure, multilayered

Table 9. Problems and Conclusions

Problem	Conclusion
Development of implants for mandibular reconstruction that are acceptable in terms of:	
– clinical requirements	Mandibular reconstruction plate
– functional stability	Condylar prosthesis
– mandibular biomechanics	Reconstruction plate with condylar head
	Anchoring element for abutment
Animal testing of the implants developed:	
Development of a suitable animal model	Minipigs, whether skeletally mature and still gaining weight or skeletally immature, that undergo resection of a 13- to 15-cm segment of the mandible without concurrent removal of the periosteum make excellent models for testing the functional soundness and stability of reconstructive procedures for extensive bone defects.
Relevance of animal experiments	The reconstruction plates are among the best-investigated implants for mandibular reconstruction in terms of defect extent, functional stability without intermaxillary fixation, and number of experimental animals.
Attainment of functional stability	The functionally stable bridging of defects can be achieved, given an appropriate operating technique.
Functional stability vs. extent of defect	Prior to our experiments there had been no animal studies on the reconstruction of a 13- to 15-cm mandibular defect without intermaxillary fixation or special dietary adjustment.
Range of application of the implants	The animal experiments are consistent with clinical experience in affirming the universal applicability of the implants, owing to their deformability in three dimensions.
Improvement of the implants	The results of animal studies and clinical experience permit ongoing improvement of the implants.
Development of corresponding operating techniques	Satisfactory anchorage of the reconstruction plates was found to affect critically the success of the reconstruction.
Operative approach	Results were equivalent with the combined intra-/extraoral approach and the purely extraoral approach.
Tissue compatibility	A correlation was noted between biocompatibility and functional stability. Investment of the implants by connective tissue was indicative of instability. When functional stability is present, the fixation screw is closely invested by bone over its entire surface.
Resistance to fracture	The implants have sufficient fracture resistance during initial bending and also after insertion, provided they are not angulated more than 15° between the plate holes.
Function of the condylar head	The bispherical transverse oval shape of the condylar head performed well by allowing unrestricted mandibular opening and preventing dislocation.

Table 9 (continued)

Problem	Conclusion
Reaction of contra-lateral joint	The contralateral joint showed no changes relative to the controls.
Placement of an abutment	The placement of an abutment (transmucosal, transalveolar, or transosseous) did not cause adverse effects in the animal experiments.
Stability of the abutment anchorage	The abutment anchorage proved to be sufficiently stable, noting that masticatory loads on the abutment were from direct contact with antagonistic teeth, since a denture was not employed.
Risk of open communication with the oral cavity	Open communication with the oral cavity appeared to have no adverse effects during the period of the animal experiments.
Epithelial margin	The presence or absence of epithelial downgrowth around the abutment depended on how stably the defect had been bridged by the implant.
Removability of the implants	Implant removability, an essential prerequisite for clinical use, was problem-free owing to the use of screw fixation and ASIF stainless steel.

closure of the oral cavity. The instrumentation for transbuccal screw insertion enables the surgeon to further curtail the extraoral phase of the procedure. Results with the bispherical, transverse oval condylar head in our animal experiments give every indication that the same design will prove favorable in clinical use. The clinical relevance of our experiments with abutments is limited, since the absence of a denture created load patterns different from those that would occur clinically.

The osseous bridging of the defect observed in our animal studies was a manifestation of functional stability and has little clinical significance beyond that, since it was a product of our experimental design (resection with preservation of the periosteum). With concurrent removal of the periosteum, which is necessary clinically in the resection of malignant tumors, bone grafting is essential in order to achieve consolidation. However, we should not discount the possibility of spontaneous bone regeneration following the subperiosteal resection of a benign neoplasm, especially in juvenile patients [4, 38, 48, 51].

Part II: Clinical Application

Materials, Methods, and Results

Since 1973, when development of the new implants began, experimental testing of the implants has been paralleled by their clinical application at the Departments of Plastic and Reconstructive Surgery of Kantonsspital Basel (Head: Prof. Dr. B. SPIESSL) until 1977 and of Inselspital Bern (Head: Prof. Dr. H. TSCHOPP) since 1978. Our clinical material is based on a follow-up of 21 consecutive cases that were operated upon between 1978 and 1982 (Inselspital Bern).

The basic case data are summarized in Table 10. Below we shall present several, more detailed case histories that serve to illustrate our experience with mandibular reconstructions.

Table 10. Outline of 21 Consecutive, Followed Cases of Mandibular Reconstruction[a]

Patient	Sex	Age (years)	Diagnosis	Implant and anchorage	Hospital stay (days)	Local complications	Implant removal (months)
1	m	28	Comminuted anterior mandibular fracture with an associated complex midfacial fracture in polytrauma from auto accident	Straight 8-hole plate, 3 screws on the right, 4 on the left	9	–	13
2	m	71	Defect of right body, angle and ramus from gunshot injury in suicide attempt	Preshaped 22-hole plate, 4 screws proximally, 6 distally	10	–	–[b]
3	m	15	Bilateral ankylosis of temporomandibular joints	Bilateral condylar prostheses, 5 screws each	6	–	–
4	m	45	Comminuted fracture of the right body with bone loss in polytrauma from auto accident	Straight 8-hole plate, 3 screws per side	8	–	–
5	f	70	Adamantinoma of the chin area	Straight 18-hole plate	5	–	–
6	m	22	Anterior mandibular defect combined with midfacial defect from gunshot injury in suicide attempt	Straight 18-hole plate, 6 screws on the right, 5 on the left	90	–	8
7	m	65	Adamantinoma of the left body and ramus	Preshaped 20-hole plate, 4 screws proximally, 6 distally	15	+[c]	4[d]
8	m	19	Comminuted anterior mandibular fracture in polytrauma from auto accident	Straight 10-hole plate, 2 screws on the right, 3 on the left	5	–	9
9	m	36	Comminuted anterior mandibular fracture with bone loss combined with midfacial disruption in polytrauma from auto accident	Straight 10-hole plate, 3 screws per side	70	+[e]	12
10	m	25	Comminuted fracture of the right angle of the mandible combined with transverse fracture of the left body, sustained in a fall	Straight 8-hole plate, 3 screws proximally, 4 distally	9	–	13
11	m	11	Sarcoma involving the left mandibular body, angle, ramus, and coronoid and condylar processes, following previous radiation and cytostatic therapy	20-hole plate with condylar head, 8 screws	15	+[f]	54[g]

12	m	42	Defect of the left mandibular angle, ramus, and condylar process combined with transverse fracture of the right body from gunshot injury in suicide attempt	16-hole plate with condylar head, 8 screws	8	—	—
13	f	40	Comminuted anterior mandibular fracture with bone loss combined with fractures of the right angle and left condylar neck in polytrauma from auto accident	Straight 6-hole plate, 2 screws on the right, 3 on the left	38	—	14
14	m	47	Comminuted fracture of the left angle with bone loss due to a fight blow (after previous resection of squamous cell carcinoma of left mesopharynx)	Straight 12-hole plate, 4 screws proximally, 5 distally	17	—[h]	—
15	m	57	Segmental fracture of the left body combined with transverse fracture of the right angle from collision during skiing	Straight 6-hole plate, 3 screws proximally, 2 distally	7	—	13
16	m	56	Comminuted fracture of the right body with bone loss	Straight 10-hole plate, 3 screws per side	6	—	18
17	m	25	Comminuted anterior fracture with bone loss from a fall during an epileptic seizure	Straight 14-hole plate, 5 screws on the right, 4 on the left	13	—	18
18	m	33	Osteomyelitis following conservative treatment of transverse fracture of the left body	Straight 10-hole plate, 4 screws on the right, 5 on the left	6	—	9
19	m	24	Comminuted anterior fracture with bone loss combined with Le Fort III fracture in polytrauma from auto accident	Straight 10-hole plate, 4 screws per side	14	+[i]	10
20	m	27	Ankylosis of the left temporomandibular joint	Left condylar prosthesis, 6 screws	15	—	—
21	m	28	Comminuted fracture of the right body in polytrauma from auto accident	Straight 12-hole plate, 4 screws proximally, 5 distally	5	—	9

[a] Performed since 1978 at the Department of Plastic and Reconstructive Surgery, Inselspital Bern. [b] Died after 2 months from other causes. [c] Plate fracture. [d] After secondary bone graft. [e] Infection in comminuted area, resolved after sequestrotomy. [f] Superficial soft-tissue infection, resolved without difficulty. [g] For secondary bone graft. [h] Died after 4½ months from carcinoma recurrence. [i] Infection in comminuted area, resolved after sequestrotomy

Case 1: A man 22 years of age was admitted with a gunshot injury of the mandible and mid-facial area. There was an anterior fracture of the mandible with bone loss and an associated skin and mucosal defect (Fig. 73a). At operation an 18-hole reconstruction plate was fitted anteriorly and attached to the mandibular stumps with 6 screws on the right side and 5 screws on the left. The defect was filled with cancellous bone taken from the iliac crest. Primary coverage was achieved by mobilizing adjacent soft tissues (Fig. 73b, c). On removal of the metal at 8 months postoperatively, good bony consolidation of the defect was noted (Fig. 73d, e).

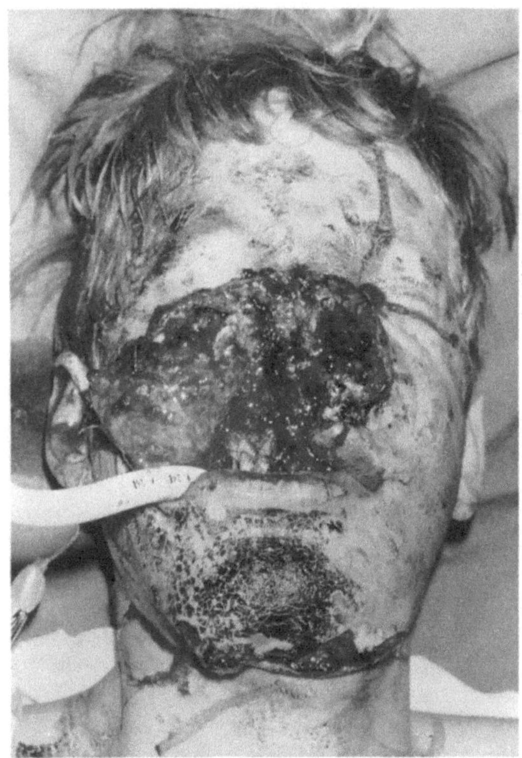

Fig. 73a–e. Case 1: 22-year-old male with gunshot injury to the mandible and midfacial region. **a** Submental entrance wound with loss of anterior bone and soft tissue. Midfacial exit wound with loss of the nose and portions of the bony maxilla

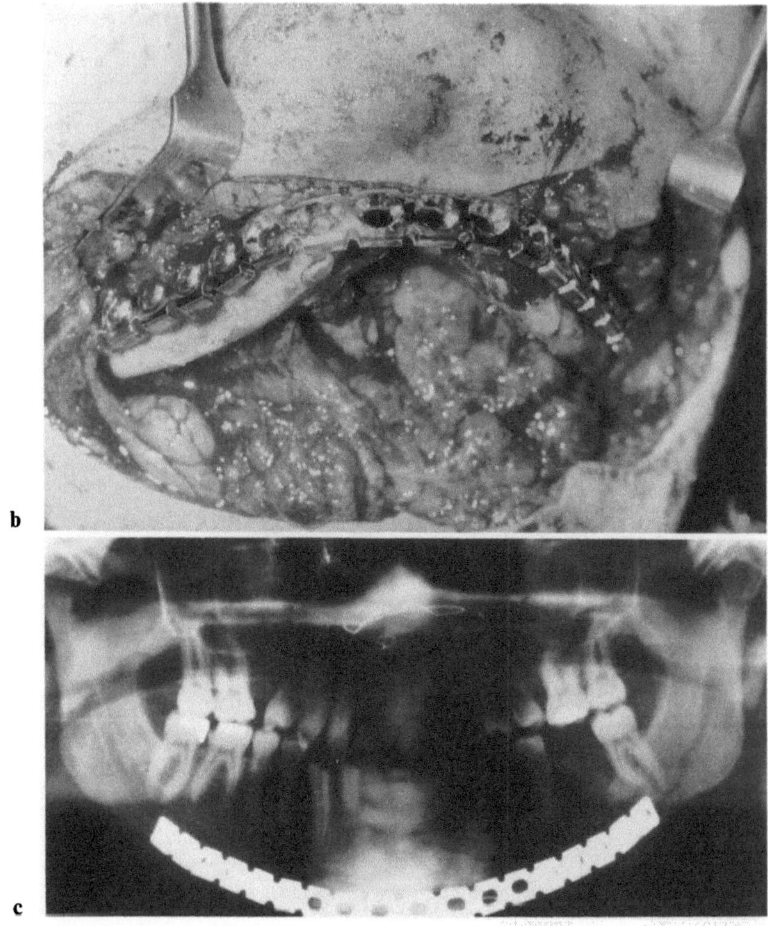

Fig. 73. **b, c** Mandibular injury was managed with an 18-hole reconstruction plate attached with 5 screws on the left side and 6 on the right and a subsequent iliac bone graft

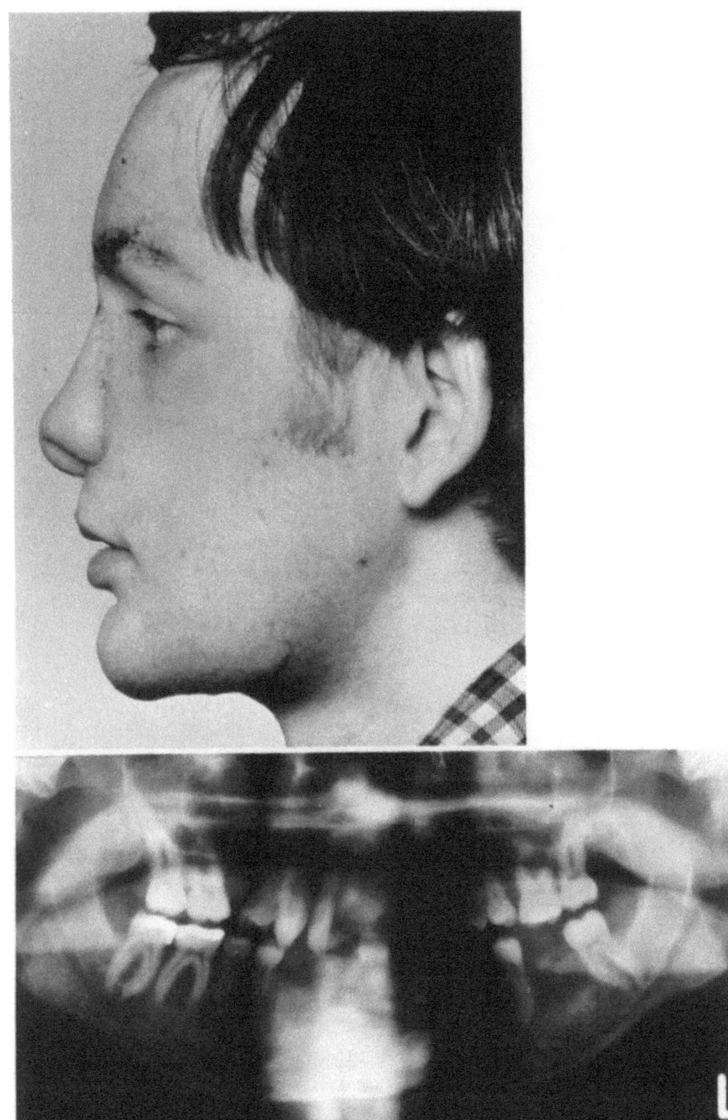

Fig. 73. d Profile appearance after bony reconstruction of the chin and nasal reconstruction with a forehead flap. **e** Roentgenogram after implant removal shows good bony consolidation of the defect

Case 2: A man 71 years of age sustained a comminuted mandibular fracture with bone loss in a gunshot injury. The mandible and tongue fell backward, causing airway obstruction (Fig. 74a). Exploration disclosed an osseous defect from the chin to the condylar neck (Fig. 74b) in addition to multiple loose bone fragments. The injury was managed with a prebent reconstruction plate. The plate was anchored with 4 screws in the articular stump and with 6 screws in the chin area (Fig. 74c). The floor of the mouth was fixed to the plate to prevent recurrence of airway obstruction. In this patient the stump of the condylar neck was barely long enough to accommodate 4 fixation screws. It is hoped that the use of special screws with expanding heads, which retain the screws in the plate holes, will make it possible to fix a short neck stump with fewer than 4 screws and still achieve a high degree of stability.

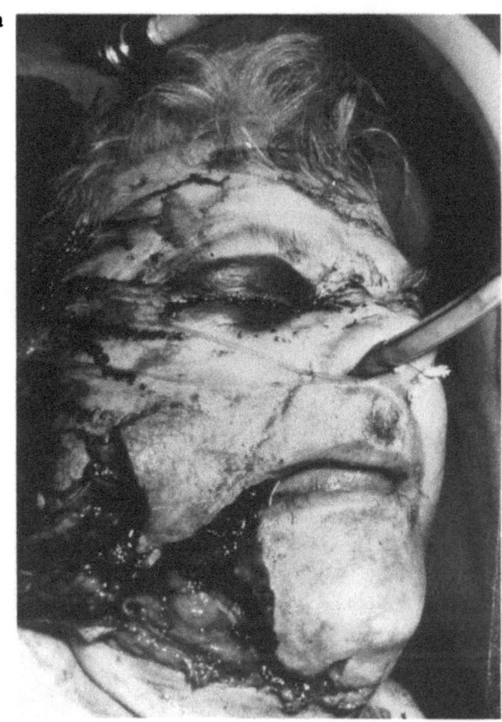

Fig. 74a – c. Case 2: 73-year-old man with gunshot injury to the right mandibular region. **a** Large cutaneous defect of the right cheek and neck. Deficient soft-tissue suspension led to airway obstruction from posterior displacement of the tongue and oral floor

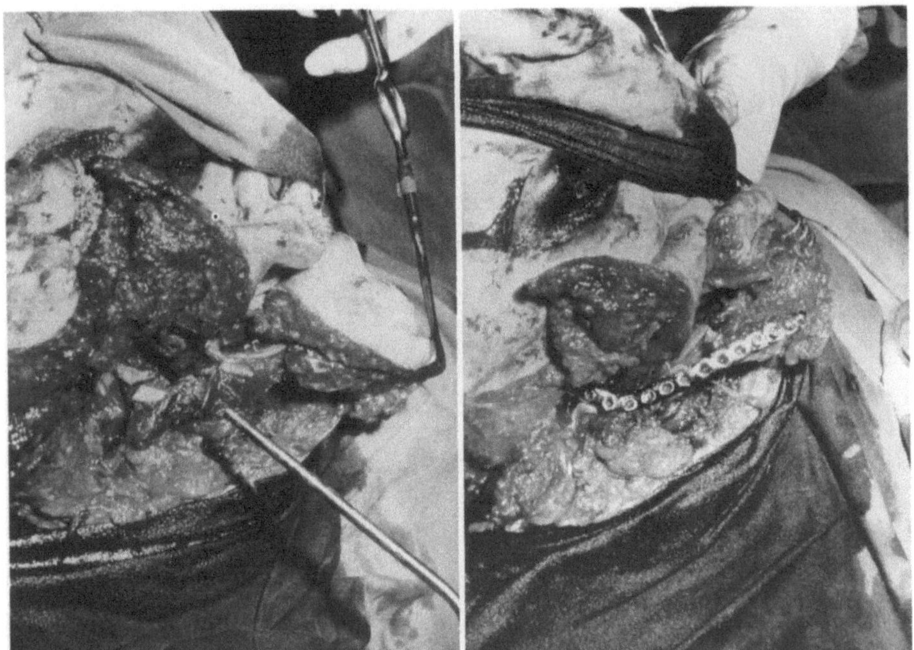

b   c

Fig. 74. b Except for a few loose bone fragments, the bony defect extends from the chin to the neck of the condyle. **c** Managed with a prebent reconstruction plate attached with 4 screws in the neck area and 6 screws in the chin area

Case 3: A 36-year-old man was involved in an auto accident, sustaning multiple midfacial fractures, a comminuted anterior mandibular fracture with bone loss, a fracture of the left condylar neck, and a Le Fort III fracture with ocular rupture in addition to fractures of the right leg. Because of the patient's poor neurologic status, consumption coagulopathy, and extreme swelling, primary treatment was limited to hemostasis, enucleation of the ruptured bulb, and tracheotomy (Fig. 75a). Postprimary treatment was started at 3 weeks after the patient's vital signs were stable and his neurologic status had improved. The mandibular stumps were fixed with a 10-hole reconstruction plate attached with 3 screws per side. Several fragments in the area of the defect were fixed with additional screws placed through the midportion of the plate and with 2 separate lag screws. Satisfactory coverage could not be obtained with adjacent tissues, and so a mucosal defect with an exposed area of bone was left on the anterior alveolar crest.

After an initially uneventful course with good granulation in the soft-tissue defect, recurrent swelling with fistula formation occurred 4 months after operation. Radiographs showed evidence of sequestration and screw loosening in the area of the defect. At 6 months the sequestra and loose screws were removed, and cancellous bone was grafted into the defect (Fig. 75b). The further course was uneventful, and stable bony bridging of the defect was noted when implant materials were removed at 12 months (Fig. 75c).

A Craniofixateur externe was used obtain functionally stable immobilization of the maxilla (Fig. 75d, e). This type of device combines well with rigid internal fixation of the mandible when a mandibular defect coexists with midfacial trauma. Early mobilization was instituted because of the coexisting condyle fracture.

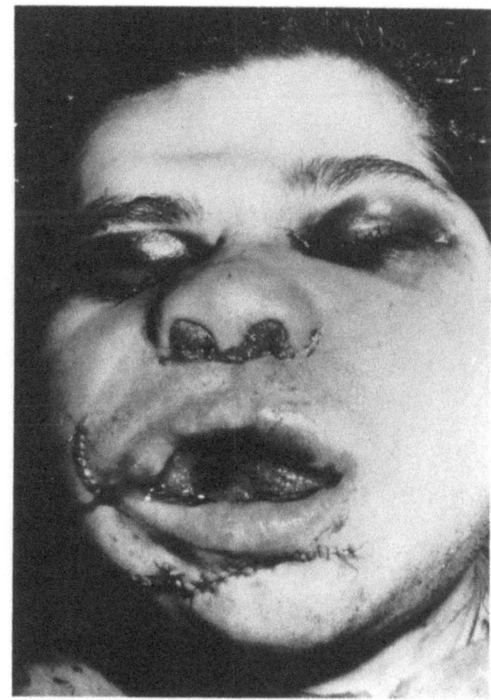

Fig. 75a–e. Case 3: 36-year-old man who sustained a comminuted anterior mandibular fracture with bone loss, a left condylar fracture, a Le Fort III fracture with midfacial comminution, and a right ocular rupture. **a** Primary care was limited to hemostasis and tamponade, enucleation of the left bulb, and tracheotomy

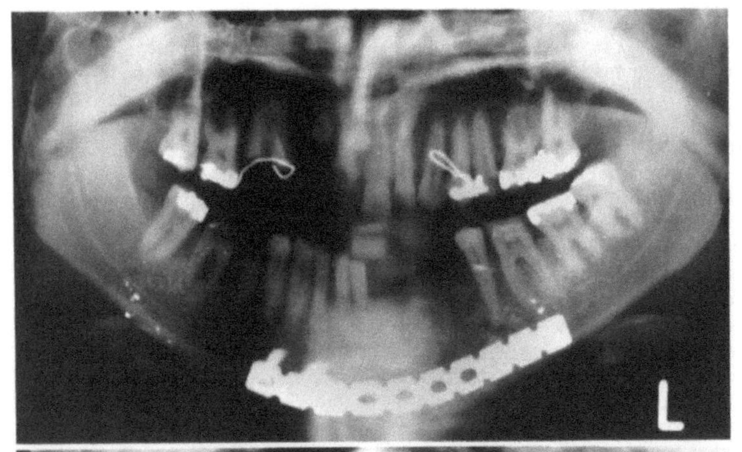

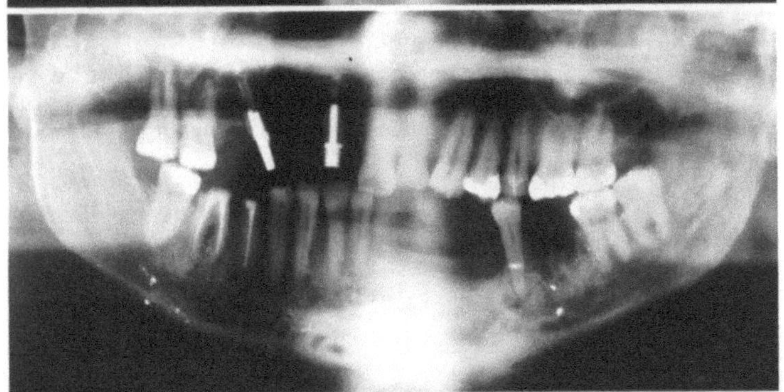

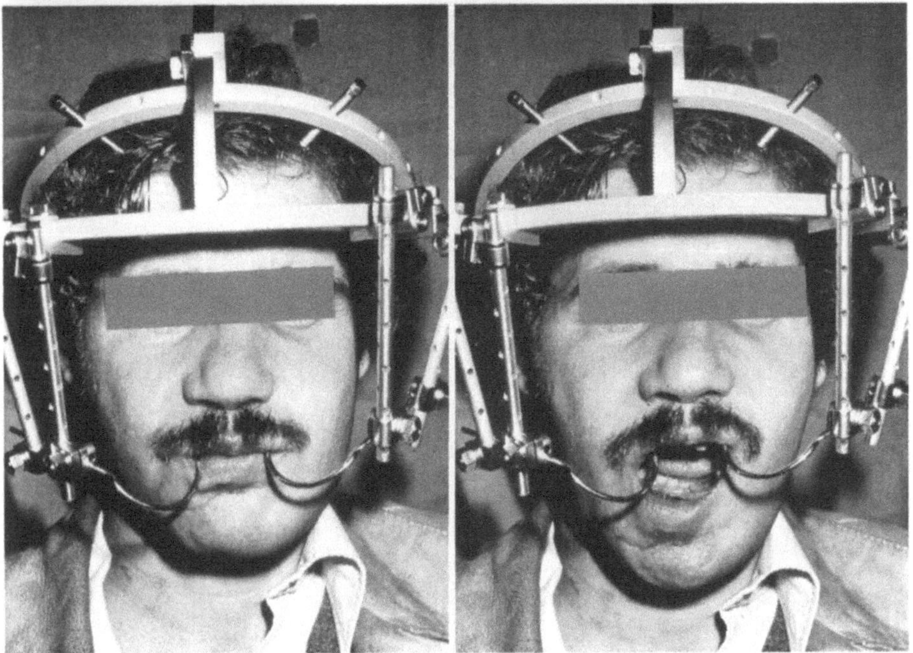

Fig. 75 b–e

Case 4: A gunshot injury in a 42-year-old man produced a fracture of the right horizontal ramus and bone loss on the left side from the mandibular angle up to and including the condyle (Fig. 76a). The right-sided fracture was managed with a 6-hole EDCP. The defect on the left side was managed with a reconstruction plate with condylar head, which was attached in the chin area with 8 screws (Fig. 76b, c). The functionally stable reconstruction obviated the need for intermaxillary fixation. Postoperative healing progressed without complications.

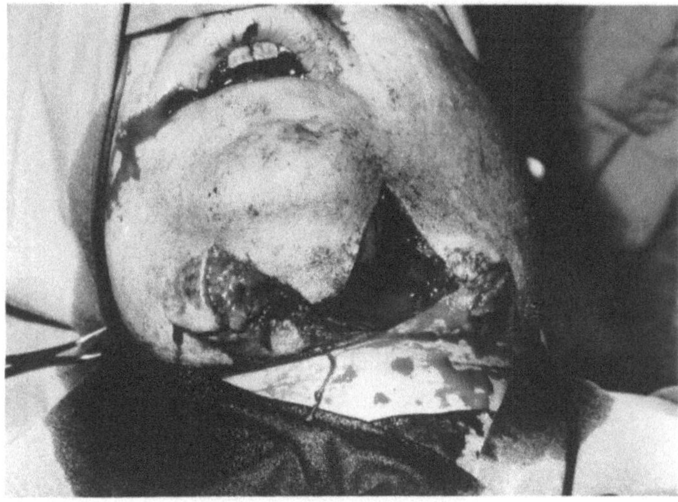

Fig. 76a – c. Case 4: 42-year-old man with gunshot injury to the left mandibular region. **a** The bullet entered through the oral floor, fracturing the right horizontal ramus of the mandible, and exited at the left ear, causing loss of the left vertical ramus and condyle.

Fig. 75. b Mandibular stumps were stabilized with a 10-hole reconstruction plate attached with 3 screws per side. Several separate lag screws for the fixation of loose fragments were removed along with sequestra after 6 months because of recurrent swelling and fistula formation, with concomitant cancellous grafting of the defect and plastic coverage of the mucosa. **c** The subsequent course was uneventful, and the jaw was well consolidated 12 months later when the implants were removed. **d, e** Maxillary injuries were stabilized with a Craniofixateur externe, which is necessary for immediate mobilization after mandibular reconstruction when combined fractures are present. Today we prefer to use the mini-reconstruction plate for this purpose. It is a miniaturized version of the standard reconstruction plate specially designed for maxillary use with 2.0-mm mini-cortex screws

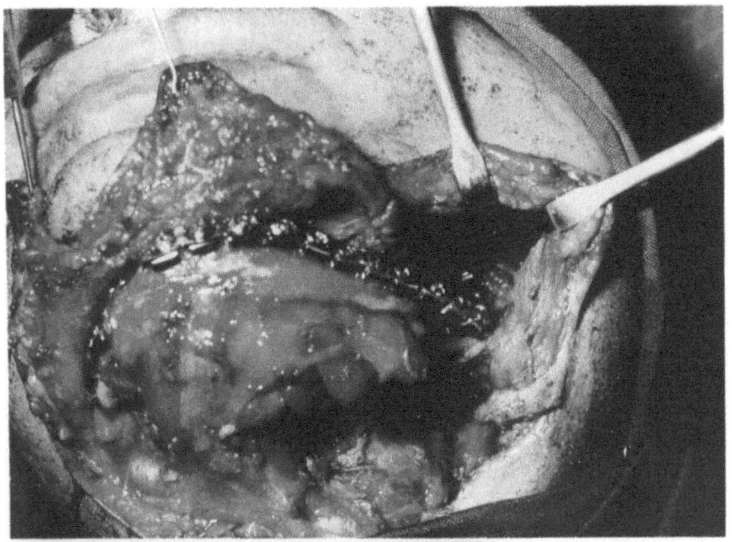

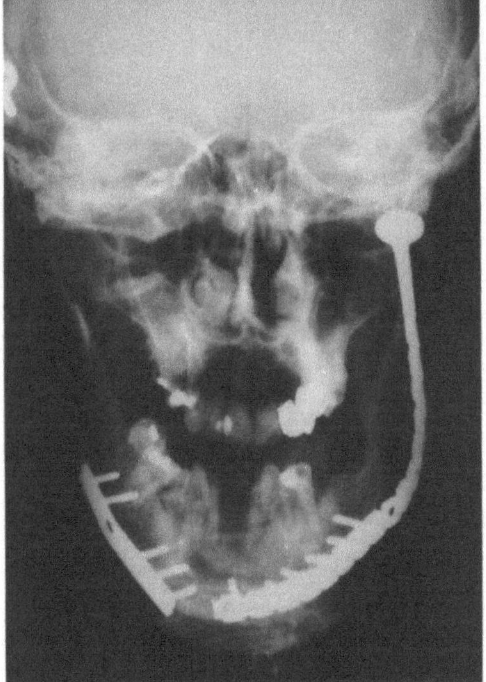

Fig. 76. b,c The fractured right horizontal ramus was managed with a 6-hole EDCP, and the left mandibular defect with a reconstruction plate with condylar head. The plate was attached in the chin area with 8 screws

Case 5: A man 65 years of age presented with a recurrent adamantinoma of the left mandibular angle that had been incompletely removed 3 years earlier. Now the tumor extended from the premolar region to the mandibular incisure and had penetrated widely into the oral cavity (Fig. 77a). The resection (Fig. 77b) and subsequent reconstruction of the mandible with a prebent 20-hole reconstruction plate were performed through an intraoral approach, using the special transbuccal instrument set (Fig. 77c) to screw the plate to the neck stump with the patient in temporary intermaxillary fixation. It was possible to place 4 screws in the neck stump and 6 screws in the chin area (Fig. 77d). The postoperative course was uneventful, and the patient could open his mouth fully with no lateral deviation of the jaw (Fig. 77e, f). Plate fracture occurred at 4 years, and the patient consented to a secondary bone graft from the iliac crest with replacement of the fractured plate. On removal of the metal 4 months later, good consolidation of the defect was confirmed.

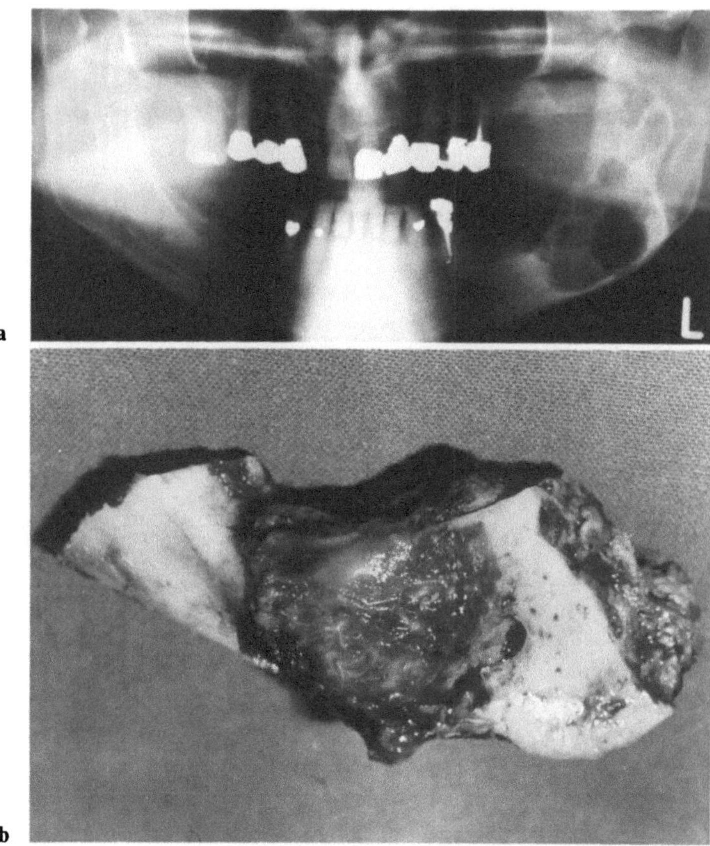

Fig. 77a–f. Case 5: 65-year-old man with recurrent adamantinoma of the left angle of the mandible. **a** Roentgenogram shows tumor involvement from the premolar region to the left semilunar incisure. **b** Resected mandibular specimen

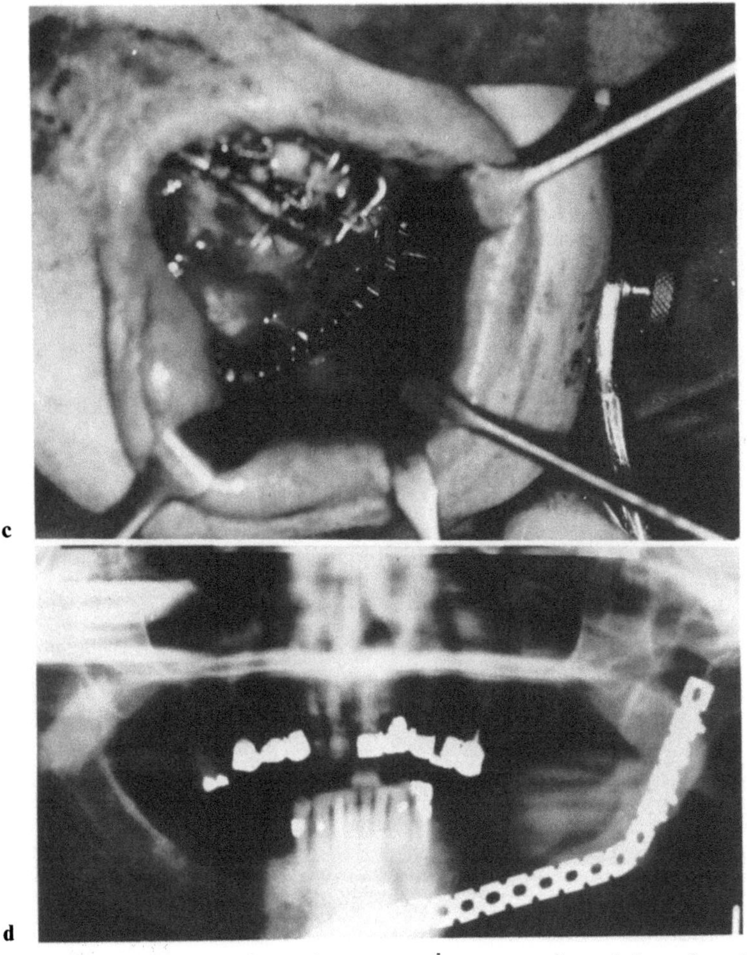

Fig. 77. c,d The resection and reconstruction were performed through an intraoral approach. The prebent 20-hole reconstruction plate was attached in the chin area with 6 screws and to the neck stump with 4 screws, which were inserted with the aid of the transbuccal instrument set

92

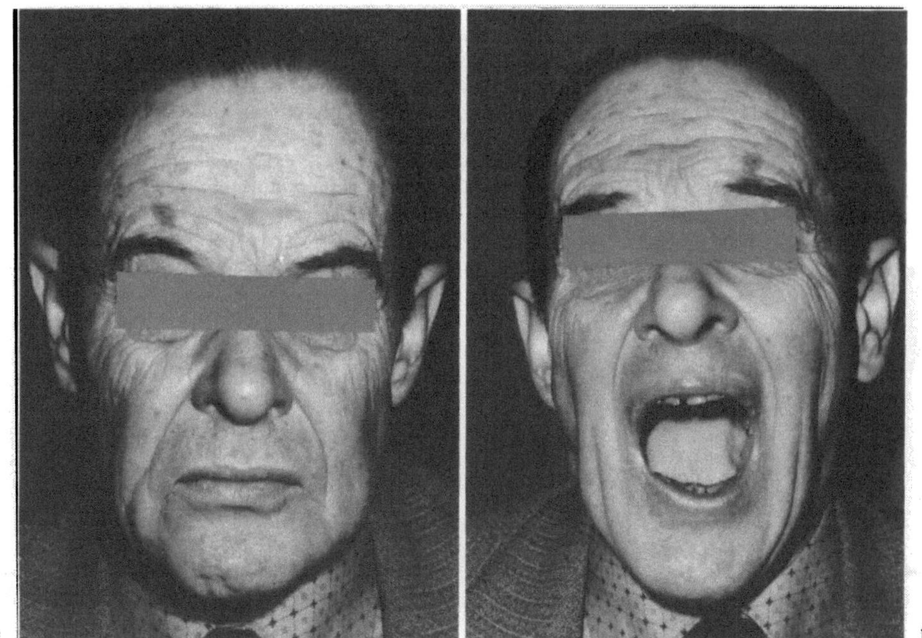

Fig. 77. e, f Mandibular opening at 3 years postoperatively is symmetrical and unrestricted

Case 6: A 15-year-old boy sustained bilateral condylar fractures of the mandible 8 years earlier, and now his maximum jaw opening is less than 10 mm (Fig. 78a). Radiographs showed
bilateral ankylosis of the temporomandibular joints. The ankylosis was resected through a
preauricular approach. Through a separate submandibular skin incision, the mandible was exposed from the horizontal ramus to the resection stump by undermining the soft tissues. With
the patient in temporary intermaxillary fixation to maintain the occlusion, a condylar prosthesis was adapted and attached on each side (Fig. 78b, c). The postoperative course was uneventful, and maximum mandibular opening 3 years after surgery exceeded 30 mm (Fig. 78d).

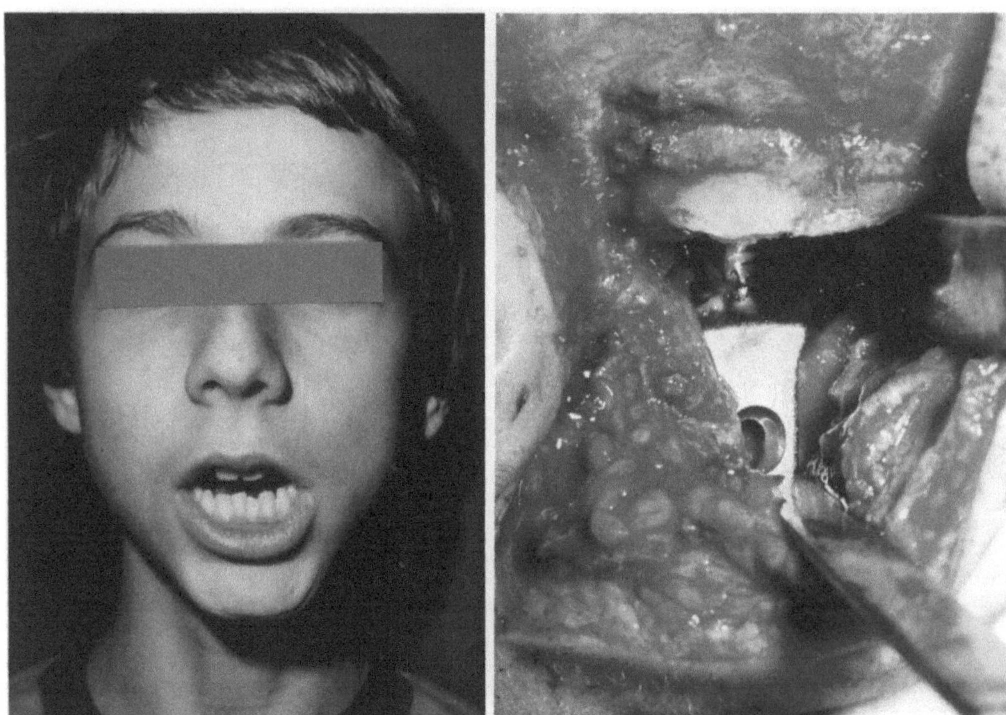

Fig. 78a–d. Case 6: 15-year-old boy with bilateral temporomandibular joint ankylosis
secondary to untreated bilateral condyle fractures at 8 years of age. **a** Maximum mandibular
opening was restricted to less than 10 mm. **b** After resecting the ankyloses and placing the
patient in temporary intermaxillary fixation to secure the occlusion, we adapted the condylar
prostheses to the mandible. When the screws are inserted, their eccentric placement relative to
the DC holes drives the spike of the prosthesis into the cancellous bone of the neck stump

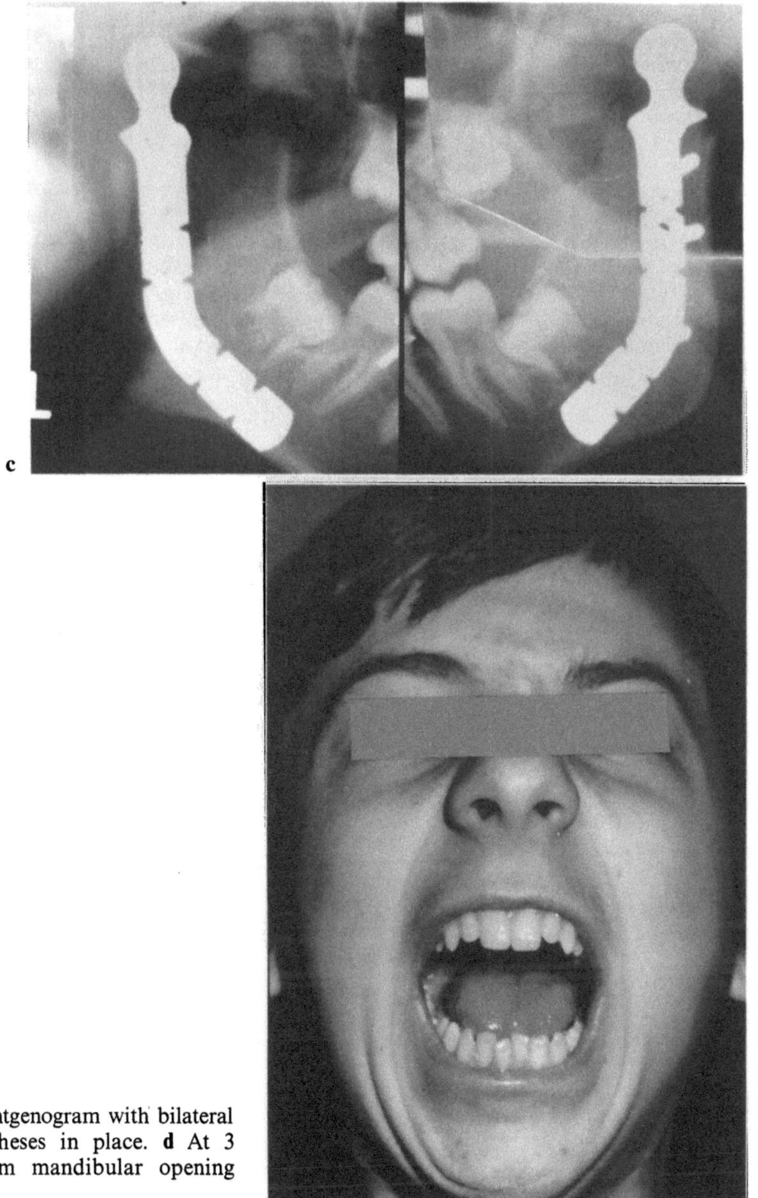

Fig. 78. c Roentgenogram with bilateral condylar prostheses in place. d At 3 years maximum mandibular opening exceeds 30 mm

Case 7: An 11-year-old boy was referred for hospitalization by his family physician because of a rapidly expanding mass in the area of the left mandibular angle. Radiographs showed an almost complete absence of bony structure from the incisure region to the articular process, so that the tooth roots appeared to be embedded in the mass (Fig. 79a). Biopsy identified the growth as a spindle-cell to polymorphocellular sarcoma. After a preliminary course of radiation and chemotherapy, the tumor was operatively removed by left hemimandibulectomy through an extraoral approach (Fig. 79b). The hemimandible was replaced by a reconstruction plate with condylar head; the head articulated with the glenoid fossa, and the distal end was attached across the midline with 8 screws (Fig. 79c). Aside from a superficial soft-tissue infection that resolved in a short time, the postoperative course was uneventful. The patient had good function with normal occlusion on the healthy side and a maximum mandibular opening greater than 45 mm without lateral deviation (Fig. 79d–f). After a recurrence-free interval of 4½ years, definitive reconstruction was accomplished with a free microvascular osteomusculocutaneous graft. Uncomplicated healing ensued, and a satisfactory morphologic and functional result was obtained.

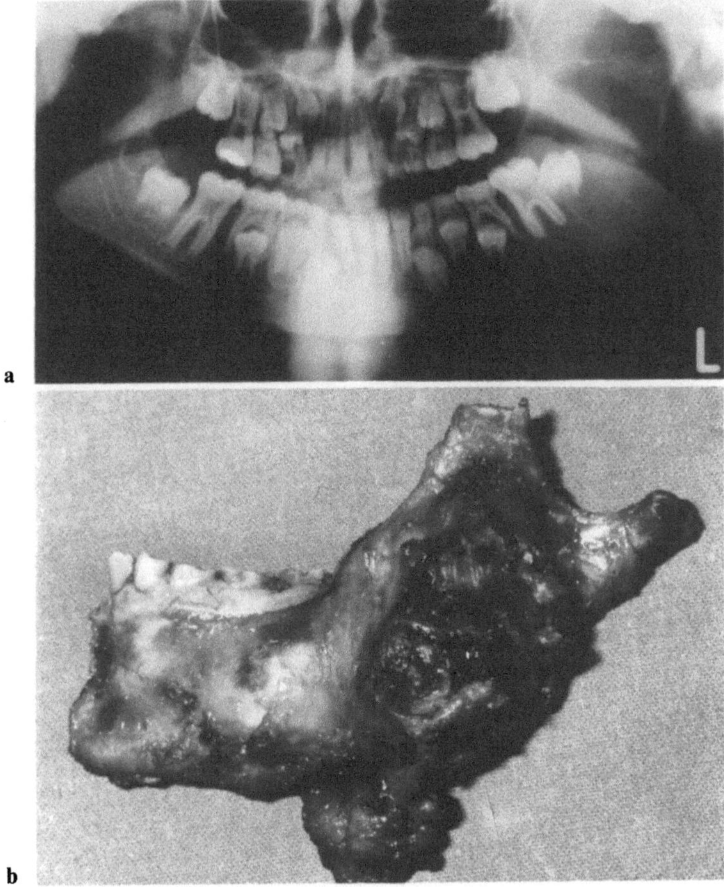

a

b

Fig. 79a, b

96

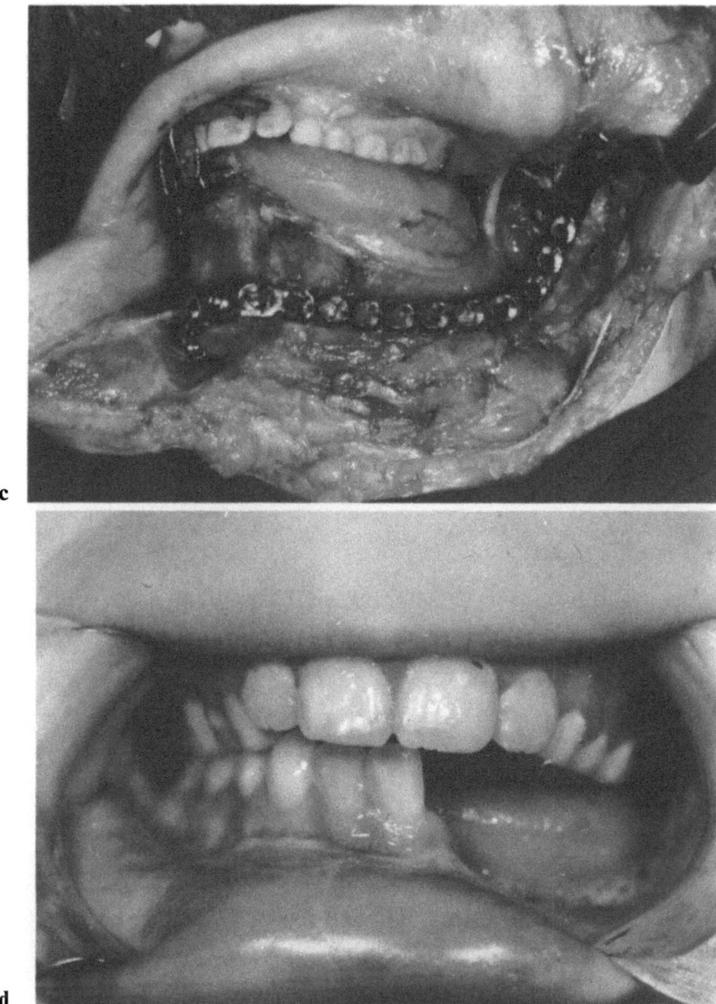

Fig. 79 a–f. Case 7: 11-year-old boy with a spindle-cell to polymorphocellular sarcoma involving the horizontal and vertical rami of the left mandible. **a** On the roentgenogram the tumor extends from the incisure area to the left coronoid and condylar processes. **b** Specimen removed at hemimandibulectomy. **c** Following the resection, we secured the right hemimandible in centric occlusion with intermaxillary fixation and reconstructed the left hemimandible with a reconstruction plate with condylar head attached across the midline with 8 screws. **d, e** One year later the mandible is symmetrical and shows correct occlusion on the right side, with a mandibular opening greater than 40 mm. The skin and mucosa are intact, even over the plate, despite damage by radiotherapy. **f** Roentgenogram of the reconstruction plate with condylar head in situ. All screws are stably anchored in the bone, and there is no evidence of bone resorption

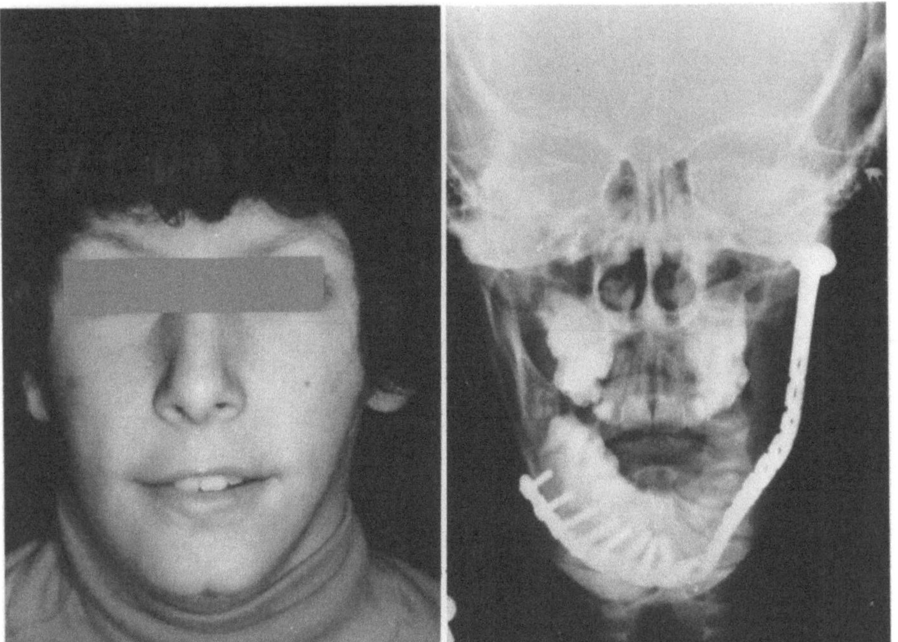

Fig. 79 e, f. (Caption see p. 97)

Discussion

In approaching the clinical problem of restoring mandibular function, our objective was to reestablish the continuity of the mandible in form, stiffness, and load-bearing ability and create a replacement for the temporomandibular joint. For this purpose implants were developed which, owing to favorable experience with rigid internal fixation of the mandible, were used clinically at the same time experimental studies were being carried out. The implants have been used in 50 patients since 1975. Thus, while the indication for the reconstruction is limited in terms of case numbers, it is frequently appropriate in severe cases, for which the procedure has proved beneficial. The present study is based on 21 mandibular reconstructions and covers only cases that have been operated and followed at our center since 1978.

Clinically, the bridging of a mandibular defect with plate fixation requires the use of at least 2 screws per side [130]. Our animal experiments demonstrated the importance of adequate stabilization. Based on these results, we try clinically to place at least 4 screws in each stump, or at least 8 screws in a free-end reconstruction. Adherence to this minimum requirement decreases the risk of delayed union, infection, and plate fracture.

Selection of an appropriate screw size was of major clinical importance. We first used screws 4.5 mm in diameter and later changed to 3.5-mm screws and

98

finally to 2.7-mm screws. The reason for this is the position of the mandibular canal, which courses an average distance of 8 mm from the mandibular border. To provide sufficient anchorage, a screw should be placed about 4 mm from the mandibular border. This leaves enough space for a maximum screw diameter of 3 mm. If the screw diameter exceeds 4 mm, there is a high probability that the screw will impinge on the nerve canal.

Either primary or secondary bone grafting may be employed in mandibular reconstructions. With a benign disorder and minimal soft-tissue damage, primary bone grafting is advised [73–78, 91]. In cases of malignancy, high-dosage radiation, or extensive soft-tissue loss, or if the patient's general condition is poor, secondary autologous bone grafts are preferred, although bone grafting is omitted in many of these cases [25, 64, 86, 118, 119, 130]. The long-term success of these procedures relies on functionally stable bridging of the bony defect. Use of the reconstruction plate for this purpose enables the early resumption of masticatory function and prevents deviation of the jaw by scar contraction [8].

The question of implant size is of crucial importance. First, it influences the attainable stabilization of the mandibular stumps; second, it plays an inhibitory role in the revascularization of bone grafts.

The transplantation of autologous bone is considered the best definitive method of mandibular reconstruction [17, 68, 128]. On the other hand, the healing of a bone graft can be the most risky phase of a mandibular reconstruction in difficult cases. A functionally stable fixation creates conditions optimum for bone graft healing, as it encourages rapid vascular ingrowth from the mandibular stump into the graft and enables the graft to remodel under a functional stimulus. Clinical experience proves that the stabilization of a bone graft with a conventional internal fixation plate on each side [130, 134] cannot be considered functionally stable. While a short, slender implant can be used on a fracture, where stabilization derives mainly from compression between the fragments, this compression is lacking during the remodeling of an interposed bone graft [115]. Presumably, remodeling processes also account for the screw loosening and frequent infection that occur within 3 months following the screw fixation of grafted bone [115]. Complications of this kind are avoidable if the bone graft can be secured by interfragmental compression. This is the purpose of the bidirectional DC holes in the mandibular reconstruction plate. It is recommended that screws in the area of the graft be removed after 3 months at the latest. The use of a one-piece graft, whether in the form of a block graft or compressed cancellous bone [17, 79], lessens the risk of nonunion in the graft area.

Experience with internal fixation of the lower extremity raises the question of whether an implant that is attached to the mandible for a period of years will produce a stress protection effect leading to loss of cortex and an increase in the proportion of cancellous bone. Clinical experience to date has shown no evidence of such an effect, even after a period of several years. However, it has been found clinically that the remodeling of a bone graft used to bridge a mandibular defect progresses more rapidly following the removal of the plate [115, 128, 131].

If a dental infection later develops in the dentulous area, retained implant material can create problems of differential diagnosis for the treating dentist. For these reasons it is desirable that the implant material be removable. The removal of a plate or the temporary loosening and reattachment of a plate may become necessary in the following cases:

— after the healing of a comminuted fracture or a fracture with bone loss
— after the healing of a bone graft
— for secondary bone grafting in which the graft is wedged between the mandibular stumps
— for reoperation due to complications (decubitus lesion, infection, etc.)
— for reoperation due to tumor recurrence
— for preprosthetic procedures
— for the insertion of a subperiosteal or endosteal implant to support a denture (e.g., a Dynamic Compression Implant [102, 106, 112, 125, 131]).

The three-dimensional bendability of the plates gives them a universal scope. The special instrument set developed for transbuccal screw fixation after sagittal split osteotomy can be used to insert implants by the intraoral route. The open communication with the oral cavity did not appear to increase the risk of infection either experimentally or clinically. The bony infections that developed in our clinical series were caused by sequestra that followed comminuted fractures. It is best to remove small, denuded bone fragments that are encountered in the area of traumatized soft tissues.

Mandibular reconstruction in patients with irradiated tumors is difficult. Bone grafts and soft tissues heal poorly under these conditions. The irradiated tissue should be replaced by healthy tissue [25, 77, 78, 91, 118, 130]. The principles of functionally stable bridging of the osseous defect still apply, although it is necessary to take certain technical precautions at operation. Poorly perfused, pedicled, or irradiated soft tissues must be absolutely free of tension when they are closed in layers over the reconstruction plate [130] because of the danger of decubitus ulcers. This should be considered at the time the plate is adapted to the jaw. The risk of decubitus can be decreased by undercontouring the plate in the endangered area [59]. The tendency to overcontour the plate should be particularly noted when adapting the plate prior to a tumor resection [130]. It is possible in principle to apply the plate to the lingual aspect of the mandible. A nut with a spherical head has been developed for fixation of the plate, although to date there has been little experience with this type of anchorage. Damaged soft tissues in the area of the implant healed well as long as stable defect bridging and tension-free wound closure were achieved.

The problem of denture attachment following an extensive mandibular resection remains largely unsolved. Preprosthetic measures can be carried out after the healing of a bone graft to facilitate the placement of a denture [86, 88], but this is a tedious undertaking that gives disappointing results in irradiated patients and patients who have had extensive flap transfers for soft-tissue coverage. The use of a Dynamic Compression Implant has been tried in such patients [131]. The prerequisite for this device is a fully integrated graft that is free of resorption and able to bear loads. The bone graft can be prepared for its future function at the time it is taken from the iliac crest [1, 13—15, 57] by inserting anchoring elements for the later attachment of abutments. The prepared graft is transplanted to the recipient bed, and after it has healed the abutments are attached. This ingenious technique also relies on a well incorporated graft with good load-bearing properties.

Our approach to the problem has been to fasten the abutments directly to the reconstruction plate via anchoring elements — a method which so far has been used only in experimental animals. The main advantage of this approach is the possibility of an absolutely stable anchorage in the residual mandibular stumps rather than in transplanted bone. The abutments may be attached without bone grafting or prior to it, or in cases where graft healing is impaired. In cases where the bone graft has become well incorporated and has borne weight for some time, it would even be possible to remove the reconstruction plate while leaving the anchoring elements and abutments in place. The anchoring elements and abutments, like the plates, can be removed without difficulty. For future clinical application after partial mandibular resections, we feel it would be safest to stabilize the jaw stumps and then wait a recurrence-free interval before proceeding with the bone graft. The risk of graft infection can be minimized by first attaching the anchoring elements by themselves and then waiting several months before inserting the abutments.

Concerning patient selection, the results in our clinical series are illuminating. The indications for the reconstruction plate consisted of fractures with comminution and bone loss, gunshot injuries, nonunions, and defects after tumor resections [109, 111, 113, 115, 127, 128, 131]. Ankylosis of the temporomandibular joint constituted a special indication for use of the condylar prosthesis. Wide resection of the ankylosed area is generally acknowledged as the treatment of choice. If a temporomandibular joint ankylosis is simply resected without interposing material at the arthroplasty site, the potential for recurrence is high [35, 39, 46, 80, 87, 94]. And without functionally stable fixation of the interposed material [20, 21, 30, 52, 54, 93, 123], a risk of dislocation exists. Therefore we consider the relatively loose interposition of a silicone block inferior to the functionally stable fixation of the condylar prosthesis [109, 116, 117, 132]. The reconstruction plate with condylar head has its major application in gunshot injuries and after tumor resections [109, 117]. There is a tendency in oncologic surgery to adopt less mutilating procedures [57] and to avoid hemimandibulectomy where possible in favor of a resection that spares the articular process. This has limited the need for the reconstruction plate with condylar head, which was used in only two of the patients in our current series. Still this does not negate the value of its development and clinical use, which was of very substantial benefit to the patients affected.

The three cases of infection in our series resulted from various causes that did not relate to lack of functional stability or tissue compatibility. Two cases had to do with small bony sequestra left after the bridging of a comminuted fracture with bone loss, and another infection developed in previously irradiated soft tissues following the reconstruction of a hemimandibulectomy for sarcoma.

Our series also included one case of plate fracture. A stable screw anchorage was found at reoperation, and so the complication probably resulted from excessive deformation of the plate when it was adapted to the mandible. Removal of the plate presented no difficulties.

In contrast to reports in the literature, we did not see complications relating to inadequate functional stability [6, 9, 12, 45] with consequent implant and screw loosening, infection, bone resorption, and migration of the implant material. We did not observe disturbances of bone graft revascularization [12, 33, 44, 45, 56, 122, 127], pressure lesions of the skin or mucosa [52, 135], or problems related to implant removal [11, 12, 16, 44, 49, 85, 93] like those variously described in the literature.

A special expanding-head screw, developed in collaboration with Mr. F. SUTTER of the Synthes Co. (Waldenburg), is currently being tested as a means of stabilizing a short mandibular neck stump with fewer than four screws. The screw head is designed to expand within the double DC hole of the reconstruction plate and stabilize it against deflection and rotation.

In the treatment of combined maxillary and mandibular fractures, functional reconstruction of the mandible must be supplemented by functionally stable fixation of the maxilla. The key to this fixation, besides the Craniofixateur externe, is the mini-reconstruction plate, which can be used to reestablish a stable load-bearing framework by restoring the four supporting pillars of the midfacial region.

Conclusions

The *development* of a reconstruction plate, an articular prosthesis, and an implant abutment which fulfill requirements in terms of load-bearing capacity, functional stability, universal applicability, tissue compatibility, and problem-free removal opens up possibilities which justify their clinical application. Discoveries made in animal experiments led to continual improvements in the implants.

The selected *experimental model* is suitable for clinically oriented investigations. As our major criteria for assessing the functional performance of the mandibular reconstruction, we selected 1) the time required to surpass weight at operation as a measure of masticatory function, 2) the occurrence of continuous bony regeneration as a measure of stability, and 3) the epithelial margin around the intraoral portion of the abutment as a measure of compatibility. Prerequisites for this model are the selection of animals that are still gaining weight (two-thirds of the studies were done in mature animals, one-third in still-growing animals) and conservation of the periosteum during resection of the bone.

With sufficient anchorage of the reconstruction plate, stability on exercise and loading (i.e., functional stability) could be achieved in mature animals as well as in animals that were still growing. The absence of intermaxillary fixation and the extent of the mandibular defect made the conditions of our animal experiments comparable to the most difficult clinical conditions.

Evaluation of the experimental study as a whole indicates that our implants can reestablish mandibular function in laboratory animals by restoring the form, stiffness, and load-bearing capacity of the mandible, by replacing the mandibular condyle, and by providing means for denture fixation; and that they perform these functions with a satisfactory degree of tisssue compatibility. The results of comparative studies in designated animal groups provide information on the minimum number of screws necessary for stable fixation, the mode of placement of abutments for denture fixation, various questions relating to operating technique, and long-term results. The good deformability of the implants ensures their *universal applicability*. The plate fracture that occurred in one patient emphasizes the importance of minimizing the amount of primary plate deformation and of awaiting further long-term results.

Both experimental and clinical observation demonstrated good *function of the joint replacement* with no adverse effects on the contralateral joint, although long-term results are again needed for a definitive assessment. So far we have not had a clinical indication for use of the implant abutments, and so no further conclusions can be drawn at present.

The animal experiments had important *clinical implications* with regard to the development and improvement of the implants and instrumentation, their handling, and refinements of operating technique. Clinical experience confirmed the experimental finding that the combined intra-/extraoral approach does not increase the incidence of infection compared with the purely extraoral approach.

The indications for clinical use of the implants were: fractures with comminution and bone loss, nonunions, gunshot injuries, defects after tumor resections, and temporomandibular joint ankylosis. Except for the ankylosis cases, we manged all osseous defects with a primary or secondary bone graft. This emphasizes the importance of problem-free removability of the implant material, which was confirmed in our experiments.

Undercontouring of the implants proved to be of crucial importance in the bridging of defects under poorly perfused or irradiated soft tissues. When conditions were stable, poorly vascularized soft tissue healed well in the area of the implant, whereas bone denuded of periosteum led to an increased risk of infection both experimentally and clinically.

On *comparing our results with previous experience,* we conclude that our implants satisfy essential requirements of bone surgery in terms of functional stability, universal applicability, use with or without bone grafting, and problem-free removal, and that they can provide a significant reduction of morbidity in patients with osseous defects of the mandible.

Acknowledgments

A great many persons contributed to the development of this work.

My first experience with the practical problems of applying new implant designs was made possible by the support of my former chief, Prof. Dr. B. SPIESSL, head of the Division of Plastic and Reconstructive Surgery of the Department of Surgery in Basel (Director: Prof. Dr. M. ALLGÖWER). My later chief, Prof. Dr. H. M. TSCHOPP, head of the Division of Plastic and Reconstructive Surgery at the Clinic for Visceral Surgery in Bern (Director: Prof. Dr. R. BERCHTOLD), aided the progress of my research with his keen interest and valuable suggestions.

The implants and instrumentation were developed in close collaboration with the manufacturer, Dr. R. MATHYS of Bettlach, and his colleague, Mr. COTTING. Both gentlemen were very receptive to all our suggestions, and their wealth of experience helped greatly in the solution of many problems.

The processing of histologic specimens was carried out under the direction of Prof. Dr. R. SCHENK, head of the Laboratory for Bone Histology of the Anatomical Institute in Bern (Director: Prof. Dr. E. WEIBEL).

The animal operations were performed at the Experimental Surgical Unit (Head: Dr. W. SCHILT), the postoperative care was administered at the Equine and Domestic Animal Clinic (Director: Prof. Dr. H. GERBER).

I am grateful to Prof. Dr. H. RIEDWYL, head of the Institute for Mathematical Statistics, for his advice on statistical evaluation.

I extend special thanks to Prof. Dr. S. M. PERREN, head of the Swiss Research Institute for Experimental Surgery in Davos and Bern, for his helpful comments concerning revisions of the manuscript.

I thank my wife for her assistance in the operations, for compling the list of references, and for taking the intraoperative and postmortem photographs. Photos of the implants were furnished by Mr. E. HUND and Mrs. M. KRETZ.

References

1. Albrektsson T, Branemark PI, Eriksson A, Lindstroem J (1978) The preformed autologous bone graft. An experimental study in rabbits. Scand J Plast Reconstr Surg 12:215
2. Allgöwer M, Perren S, Matter P (1970) A new plate for internal fixation — The Dynamic Compression Plate (DCP). Injury 2:40
3. Allgöwer M, Kinzl L, Matter P, Perren S, Rüdi T (1973) Die Dynamische Kompressionsplatte DCP. Springer, Berlin Heidelberg New York
4. Anastassov K, Popov K (1975) Régénération complète du corps de la branche montante et du condyle de la mandibule chez un enfant après désarticulation. Rev Odontostomatol (Paris) 4:43
5. Anderson R (1958) Prosthetic replacement of the hemisected mandible. Cleve Clin Q 25:18
6. Austermann KH, Becker R, Bruning K, Machtens E (1977) Titanium implants as a temporary replacement of mandible. A report of 30 cases. J Maxillofac Surg 5:167
7. Becker R, Machtens E (1972) Temporärer Ersatz des Unterkiefers. 1. Kongreß der Europäischen Gesellschaft für Kiefer- und Gesichtschirurgie. 28. Sept.—1. Okt. 1972, Ljubliana
8. Bergenfeldt E (1929) Prothesenbehandelter Fall nach halbseitiger Unterkieferexartikulation wegen Adamantinom, nebst einer kurzen Übersicht über die Behandlungsmethoden für Ersatz von Unterkieferdefekten. Acta Chir Scand 64:473
9. Bowerman JE (1974) A review of reconstruction of the mandible. Proc R Soc Med 67:610
10. Bowerman JE, Conroy B (1969) An universal kit in titanium for immediate replacement of the resected mandible. Br J Oral Surg 6:223
11. Boyne PJ (1969) Restoration of osseous defects in maxillofacial casualties. J Am Dent Assoc 78:767
12. Boyne PJ, Zarem H (1976) Osseous reconstruction of the resected mandible. Am J Surg 132:49
13. Branemark PI, Breine U, Hallen O, Hanson B, Lindstroem J (1970) Repair of defects in mandible. Scand J Plast Reconstr Surg 4:100
14. Branemark PI, Lindström J, Hallen O, Breine U, Jeppson PH, Öhman A (1975) Reconstrution of the defective mandible. Scand J Plast Reconstr Surg 9:116
15. Breine U, Branemark PI (1980) Reconstruction of alveolar jaw bone. An experimental and clinical study of ediate and preformed bone grafts in combination with osseointegrated implants. Scand J Plast Reconstr Surg 14:23
16. Brown KE (1971) Supportive metallic implant for autogenous mandibular graft. J Prosthet Dent 26:205
17. Burri C, Wolter D (1977) Das komprimierte autologe Spongiosatransplantat. Unfallheilkunde 80:169
18. Casson PR, Eitches A, Hayes CW (1972) Reconstruction of the mandible by iliac bone grafting. International symposium on plastic and reconstructive surgery of the face and neck. Aesthetic Plast Surg 1:220
19. Casterman A, Garsse A van, Vanwijck R (1977) Primary reconstruction of the mandible after resection for oral cancer. Acta Chir Belg 76:205
20. Castigliano SG, Gross PP (1951) Immediate prosthesis following radical resection in advanced primary malignant neoplasm of the mandible. J Oral Surg 9:31
21. Catania VC, Cislaghi E, Bandettini MV (1970) Immediate replacement with metal prosthesis of hemimandible removed for neoplasia. Minerva Stomatol 19:433

22. Cernea P, Crepy C, Benoist M (1966) Reconstruction mandibulaire immédiate après résection. Mém Acad Chir 92:66
23. Cole PP (1918) Ununited fractures of the mandible; their incidence, causation, and treatment. Br J Surg 6:57
24. Conley JJ (1951) The use of vitallium prostheses and implants in the reconstruction of the mandibular arch. Plast Reconstr Surg 8:150
25. Conley JJ (1953) A technique of immediate bone grafting in the treatment of benign and malignant tumors of the mandible and a review of seventeen consecutive cases. Cancer 6:568
26. Conley JJ (1956) Management of tumors of the inferior alveolar process and mandible with special emphasis on immediate bone grafting. J Oral Surg 14:325
27. Conley JJ, Pack GT (1949) Surgical treatment of malignant tumors of the inferior alveolus and mandible. Arch Otolaryngol 50:513
28. Converse JM, Campbell RM (1950) Experiences with a bone bank in plastic surgery. Plast Reconstr Surg 5:258
29. Converse JM, Shapiro HH (1954) Bone grafting in malformations of the jaws. Am J Surg 88:858
30. Cook HP (1968) Immediate reconstruction of the mandible by metallic implant following resection for neoplasm. Ann R Coll Surg Engl 42:233
31. Danis R (1949) Théorie et pratique de l'ostéosynthèse. Paris, Masson
32. Deaderick WH (1823) Case of removal of a portion of the lower maxillary bone. Am Med Rec 6:516
33. Dechamplain RQ (1973) Mandibular reconstruction. J Oral Surg 31:448
34. Duker J, Haerle F, Niederdellmann H (1976) Beckenspantransplantat im Unterkiefer unter belastungsstabilen Verhältnissen im Tierexperiment. Fortschr Kiefer Gesichtschir 20:21
35. Estabrooks LN, Murnane TW, Doku HC (1972) The role of condylotomy with interpositional silicone rubber in temporo-mandibular joint ankylosis. Oral Surg 34:2
36. Flinchbaugh RW (1958) Prostodontic aspects of an implant for hemimandible. J Prosthet Dent 8:1039
37. Fordyce GL (1971) A new method for the reconstruction of the body of the mandible following resection for recurrent adamantinoma. Br J Oral Surg 8:237
38. Francksen U (1958) Periostale Regeneration des Unterkiefers nach halbseitiger Exartikulation. Fortschr Kiefer Gesichtschir 4:337
39. Freedman GL, Gordon RL (1968) Unilateral bony ankylosis of the temporo-mandibular joint: report of case. J Oral Surg 26:807
40. Freeman BS (1948) The use of vitallium plates to maintain function following resection of the mandible. Plast Reconstr Surg 3:73
41. Gaisford JC, Hanna DC, Gutman D (1961) Management of the mandibular fragments following resection. Plast Reconstr Surg 28:192
42. Gaskins JA Jr, Ertugrul G, Rush BF Jr (1969) Tolerance to stainless steel prostheses in patients after postradiation hemimandibulectomy. Am J Surg 117:375
43. Gräfe CF von (1821) Herausnahme der halben Unterkinnlade mit ihrem Gelenkkopfe und die dazu notwendige Unterbindung der Carotis an der linken Seite des Halses am Kehlkopfe. Allg Med Ann (Leipzig) 1143
44. Hahn GW (1964) Vitallium mesh mandibular prosthesis. J Prosthet Dent 14:777
45. Hahn GW, Corgill DA (1969) Chrome cobalt mesh mandibular prosthesis. J Oral Surg 27:5
46. Hartwell SW Jr, Hall MD (1974) Mandibular condylectomy with silicone rubber replacement. Plast Reconstr Surg 53:440
47. Hauenstein H, Steinhäuser EW (1977) Erfahrungen mit dem Titan-Gitter als temporäres Fremdimplantat zur Wiederherstellung bei Unterkieferdefekten. Dtsch Zahnarztl Z 32:523
48. Haunfelder D (1962) Über die Regeneration des Unterkiefers nach subperiostaler Resektion und Exartikulation. Chirurg 33:62
49. Heidsieck C (1961) Entfernung gutartiger Kiefertumoren und osteoplastische Defektdeckung bei enoralem Vorgehen. Fortschr Kiefer Gesichtschir 7:198

50. Heidsieck C (1978) Fixation of the edentulous residual portion of the mandible in cases of hemimandibulectomy. J Maxillofac Surg 6:21
51. Kazanjian VH (1946) Spontaneous regeneration of bone following excision of section of the mandible. Am J Orthod 32:242
52. Kleitsch WP (1951) Vitallium reconstruction of a hemimandible and temporo-mandibular joint. Plast Reconstr Surg 7:244
53. Krompecher G (1937) Die Knochenbildung. Fischer, Jena
54. Lane SL, Hoffman B, Lane JV (1958) Vitallium implant for transsected portion of the mandible. Am J Surg 96:768
55. Lathouwer C de, Lernick PL, Mayer R, Mendes P (1974) Deux cas de sarcome ostéogénique de la mandibule. Intérêt de la reconstruction immédiate. Acta Chir Belg 73:49
56. Lewis JD (1971) Prothèse grillagées en vitallium dans la reconstruction de la mandibule. Rev Stomatol Chir Maxillofac 72:290
57. Lindström J, Branemark IP, Albrektsson T (1981) Mandibular reconstruction using the preformed autologous bone graft. Scand J Plast Reconstr Surg 15:29
58. Luhr HG (1976) Ein Plattensystem zur Unterkieferrekonstruktion einschließlich des Gelenkersatzes. Dtsch Zahnarztl Z 31:747
59. Luhr HG (1978) Der freie Unterkieferersatz – Berücksichtigung des Transplantatlagers bei der Rekonstruktion. Fortschr Kiefer Gesichtschir 23:48
60. Mac Dougall JA (1965) Management of surgical mandibular defects. Am J Surg 110:562
61. Manchester WM (1972) Some technical improvements in the reconstruction of the mandible and temporo-mandibular joint. Plast Reconstr Surg 50:249
62. Masson JK (1965) A variation of Kirschner wire prosthesis for reconstruction of mandible after partial mandibular resection for intraoral malignancy. Plast Reconstr Surg 35:457
63. Mc Quarrie DG (1968) Reconstruction of the mandible with a simple prosthesis at the time of radical surgery for oral carcinoma. Report of thirteen cases. Lancet 88:282
64. Millard DR Jr (1964) A new approach to immediate mandibular repair. Ann Surg 160:306
65. Millard DR Jr, Deane M, Garst WP (1971) Bending an iliac bone graft for anterior mandibular arch repair. Plast Reconstr Surg 48:600
66. Mladick RA, Horton CE, Adamson JE, Carraway J (1972) A simple technique for securing a K-wire to the mandible. Plast Reconstr Surg 49:228
67. Momma WG (1977) Erste Ergebnisse mit einem alloplastischen Kiefergelenkersatz einschließlich Pfanne. Dtsch Zahnarztl Z 32:326
68. Mowlem R (1944) Cancellous chip bone-grafts. Report on 75 cases. Lancet 2:746
69. Müller ME, Allgöwer M, Willenegger H (1963) Technik der operativen Frakturenbehandlung. Springer, Berlin Göttingen Heidelberg
70. Müller ME, Allgöwer M, Willenegger H (1969) Manual der Osteosynthese. Springer, Berlin Heidelberg New York
71. Müller ME, Allgöwer M, Schneider R, Willenegger H (1977) Manual der Osteosynthese, 2. Aufl. Springer, Berlin Heidelberg New York
72. Nasteff D (1958) Intraorale Kieferresektion. Zahnaerztliche Praxis 9:18
73. Obwegeser H (1960) Aktives chirurgisches Vorgehen bei der Osteomyelitis mandibulae. Oesterr Z Stomatol 57:216
74. Obwegeser H (1963) Probleme und Möglichkeiten der Unterkieferresektion und gleichzeitigen Rekonstruktion auf dem oralen Operationswege. Schweiz Monatsschr Zahnheilkd 73:830
75. Obwegeser H (1965) Erfahrungen der einzeitigen Unterkieferresektion und -rekonstruktion auf dem oralen Operationswege. Oesterr Z Stomatol 62:261
76. Obwegeser HL (1966) Simultaneous resection and reconstruction of parts of the mandible via the intraoral route in patients with and without gross infections. Oral Surg 21:693
77. Obwegeser HL (1968) Primary repair of the mandible by the intraoral route after partial resection in cases with and without pre-operative infection. Br J Plast Surg 21:282
78. Obwegeser HL, Sailer HF (1978) Experiences with intraoral partial resection and simultaneous reconstruction in cases of mandibular osteomyelitis. J Macillofac Surg 6:34

79. Osborn JF, Spiessl B (1980) Herstellung und Eigenschaften druckgeformter Spongiosatransplantate. Dtsch Zahnarztl Z 35:1924
80. Parmer DE, Pederson GW (1972) Arthroplasty for bilateral temporo-mandibular joint ankylosis: report of case. J Oral Surg 30:816
81. Perren S, Huggler M, Russenberger M et al. (1969a) The reaction of cortical bone to compression. Acta Orthop Scand [Suppl] 125:17
82. Perren SM, Hutzschenreuter P, Steinemann S, Geret V, Klebel M (1969b) Some effects of rigidity of internal fixation on the healing pattern of osteotomies. Injury 1:77
83. Pickerill HP (1918) Methods of control of fragments in gunshot wounds of the jaws. Lancet 2:313
84. Rahn BA (1976) Die polychrome Sequenzmarkierung. Habilitationsschrift, Universität Freiburg/Br
85. Raveh J, Stich H, Sutter F, Schachwalder P (1981) Neue Rekonstruktionsmöglichkeiten bei Unterkieferdefekten nach Tumorresektion. Schweiz Mschr Zahnheilkd 91:899
86. Rehrmann A (1956) Autoplastic reconstruction; technic for avoiding facial nerve and vascular injuries. Plast Reconstr Surg 17:452
87. Rehrmann A (1967) Eine Methode zur operativen Beseitigung der doppelseitigen Ankylose der Kiefergelenke durch breite Knochenresektion, temporäre Implantation von Palavitkörpern und autogene Knochentransplantation. Fortschr Kiefer Gesichtschir 12:64
88. Rehrmann A (1978) Das freie Knochentransplantat zum Unterkieferersatz unter besonderer Berücksichtigung der Kinnrekonstruktion. Fortschr Kiefer Gesichtschir 23:39
89. Reuther JF (1977) Druckplattenosteosynthese und freie Knochentransplantation zur Unterkieferrekonstruktion. Experimentelle und klinische Untersuchungen. Habilitationsschrift, Universität Mainz
90. Reuther JF, Hausamen JE (1977) System zur alloplastischen Überbrückung von Unterkieferdefekten. Dtsch Zahnarztl Z 32:334
91. Sailer HF (1976) Ergebnisse der gleichzeitigen Resektion und Rekonstruktion des Unterkiefers auf oralem Weg. Fortschr Kiefer Gesichtschir 20:45
92. Sako K, Marchetta FC (1962) The use of metal prostheses following anterior mandibulectomy and neck dissection for carcinoma of the oral cavity. Am J Surg 104:715
93. Salyer KE, Newsom HT, Holmes R, Hahn G (1977) Mandibular reconstruction. Am J Surg 134:461
94. Sanders B, Brady FA, Adams D (1977) Silastic cap temporo-mandibular joint prosthesis. J Oral Surg 35:933
95. Schenk RK (1965) Zur histologischen Verarbeitung von unentkalkten Knochen. Acta Anat (Basel) 60:3
96. Schenk BK, Willenegger H (1963) Zum histologischen Bild der sogenannten Primärheilung der Knochenkompakta nach experimentellen Osteotomien am Hund. Experienta 19:593
97. Schenk RK, Willenegger H (1964) Histologie der primären Knochenheilung. Langenbecks Arch Chir 308:440
98. Schenk RK, Willenegger H (1967) Morphological findings in primary fracture healing. Symp Biol Hung 7:75
99. Schmelzle R, Schwenzer N (1976) Ein neuer Plattentyp zur Defektüberbrückung nach Unterkieferresektion (Tübinger Unterkieferresektions-Platte). Dtsch Zahnarztl Z 31:819
100. Schmoker R (1973) Exzentrisch dynamische Kompressionsplatte sowie Kompressionszuggurtungsschiene, Kompressionszuggurtungsplatte und Repositionskompressionszange. Eine neue Technik der funktionsstabilen Unterkieferosteosynthese mit Kompression auf der Zugseite, Dissertation, Universität Basel
101. Schmoker R (1975a) Experimentelle Untersuchungen zur Stabilität und intraoperativen Kompression bei der Osteosynthese von Unterkieferfrakturen. AO-Bulletin
102. Schmoker R (1975b) Experimentelle Untersuchungen zur Stabilität des funktionsstabilen Gerüstimplantates. Schweiz Monatsschr Zahnheilkd 85:154
103. Schmoker R (1975c) Zur Operationsplanung bei Progenie und Retrogeniefällen. Schweiz Monatsschr Zahnheilkd 85:598
104. Schmoker R (1976a) The Eccentric Dynamic Compression Plate. An experimental study as to it's contribution to the functionally stable internal fixation of fractures of the lower

jaw. AO-Bulletin. Official Pulication of the Swiss Association for the Study of Internal Fixation (ASIF)

105. Schmoker R (1976 b) Experimental studies on the effect of rigidity using an Eccentric Dynamic Compression Plate (EDCP). In: Spiessl B (ed) New concepts in maxillofacial bone surgery. Springer, Berlin Heidelberg New York, p 41

106. Schmoker R (1976 c) Experimental studies on the stability of the Dynamic Compression Implant. In: Spiessl B (ed) New concepts in maxillofacial bone surgery. Springer, Berlin Heidelberg New York, p 144

107. Schmoker R (1976 d) Internal fixation of mandibular fractures using an Eccentric Dynamic Compression Plate (ECDP). In: Spiessl B (ed) New concepts in maxillofacial bone surgery. Springer, Berlin Heidelberg New York, p 53

108. Schmoker R (1976 e) Preoperative planning of sagittal split osteotomy of the ascending mandibular ramus (simulography). In: Spiessl B (ed) New concepts in maxillofacial bone surgery. Springer, Berlin Heidelberg New York, p 98

109. Schmoker R (1983) Rigid internal fixation of compound fractures of the mandible using a specially designed reconstruction plate. First International Symposium on Maxillofacial Trauma, Nov. 13−15, 1981, Detroit. In: Jacobs JR (ed) Maxillofacial trauma: an international perspective. Praeger, New York, p 187

110. Schmoker R, Tschopp HM (1979 a) Präoperative Planung der sagittalen Spaltungsosteotomie mittels Simulographie. Dtsch Z Mund Kiefer Gesichtschir 3:37

111. Schmoker R, Tschopp HM (1979 b) Prinzipien zur Versorgung von Gesichtsfrakturen. Helv Chir Acta 46:39

112. Schmoker R, Cornioley D, Huser W, Spiessl B, Graf H (1976 a) Experimental studies of the load-bearing properties of implanted prostheses. In: Spiessl B (ed) New concepts in maxillofacial bone surgery. Springer, Berlin Heidelberg New York, p 141

113. Schmoker R, Spiessl B, Mathys R (1976 b) A total mandibular plate to bridge large defects of the mandible. In: Spiessl B (ed) New concepts in maxillofacial bone surgery. Springer, Berlin Heidelberg New York, p 156

114. Schmoker R, Eulenberger J, Spiessl B, Mathys R (1977 a) Entwicklung und tierexperimentelle Untersuchung einer Kieferköpfchenprothese. Dtsch Z Mund Kiefer Gesichtschir 1:86

115. Schmoker R, Spiessl B, Mathys R (1977 b) Eine Rekonstruktionsplatte zur Überbrückung größerer Knochendefekte im Unterkiefer. Aktuel Traumatol 7:199

116. Schmoker R, Tschopp HM, Allmen G von (1979) Korrekturoperationen bei Spätfolgen nach Gesichtsschädelfrakturen. Gemeinsame Tagung der Schweizerischen und Österreichischen Gesellschaft für Plastische und Wiederherstellungschirurgie. 12.−15. 9. 1979, Luzern

117. Schmoker R, Allmen G von, Tschopp HM (1981) Der künstliche Ersatz des Kiefergelenks. Schweiz Monatsschr Zahnheilkd 91:222

118. Schröder F (1967) Spätplastik und Sofortplastik nach Unterkieferresektion. Dtsch Zahn Mund Kieferheilkd 48:1

119. Schröder F (1979) Kinnrekonstruktion nach Tumorresektion. Fortschr Kiefer Gesichtschir 24:98

120. Schröder A, Pohler O, Sutter F (1976) Gewebsreaktion auf ein Titan-Hohlzylinderimplantat mit Titan-Spritzschichtoberfläche. Schweiz Monatsschr Zahnheilkd 86:713

121. Schröder A, Zypen E van der, Stich H, Sutter F (1981) The reactions of bone, connective tissue and epithelium to endosteal implants with titanium sprayed surfaces. J Maxillofac Surg 9:15

122. Seymour RL, Bray TE, Irby WB (1977) Replacement of condylar process. J Oral Surg 35:405

123. Silver CM, Motamed M, Carlotti AE Jr (1977) Arthroplasty of the temporo-mandibular joint with use of a vitallium condyle prosthesis: report of three cases. J Oral Surg 35:909

124. Skaloud F (1953) Die Überbrückung von Unterkieferdefekten und Fixation von Bruchstücken durch Metallnagelung bei Mandibularresektionen. Dtsch Zahn Mund Kieferheilkd 19:36

125. Spiessl B (1974) Die funktionsstabile Implantatprothese. Theoretische und praktische Grundlagen. Schweiz Monatsschr Zahnheilkd 84:726

126. Spiessl B (1976) Erste Erfahrungen mit einer Kiefergelenksprothese. Fortschr Kiefer Gesichtschir 21:119
127. Spiessl B (1978) Die Unterkiefer-Resektionsplatte der AO. Ihre Anwendung bei Unterkieferdefekten in der Tumorchirurgie. Unfallheilkund 81:389
128. Spiessl B (1981) A new method of anatomical reconstruction of extensive defects of the mandible with autogenous cancellous bone. J Maxillofac Surg 8:78
129. Spiessl B, Schroll K (1972) Gesichtsschädel, Bd I/1. In: Nigst H (Hrsg) Spezielle Frakturen- und Luxationslehre. Thieme, Stuttgart
130. Spiessl B, Tschopp HM (1974) Chirurgie der Kiefer. In: Naumann H (Hrsg) Kopf- und Hals-Chirurgie, Bd 2/2: Gesicht und Gesichtsschädel. Thieme, Stuttgart, p 683
131. Spiessl B, Prein J, Schmoker R (1976a) Anatomical reconstruction and functional rehabilitation of mandibular defects after ablative surgery. In: Spiessl B (ed) New concepts in maxillofacial bone surgery. Springer, Berlin Heidelberg New York, p 160
132. Spiessl B, Schmoker R, Mathys R (1976b) Treatment of ankylosis by a condylar prosthesis of the mandible. In: Spiessl B (ed) New concepts in maxillofacial bone surgery. Springer, Berlin Heidelberg New York, p 83
133. Steinhäuser E (1968) Unterkieferrekonstruktion durch intraorale Knochentransplantate, deren Einheilung und Beeinflussung durch die funktions- und tierexperimentelle Studie (Teil I, II). Schweiz Monatsschr Zahnheilkd 78:213
134. Stellmach R (1978) Die Fixierung des Spans bei der freien Knochentransplantation. Fortschr Kiefer Gesichtschir 23:58
135. Tarnai K (1954) Operative Metallallenthese-Implantation in einer Sitzung zum Ersatz des fehlenden Unterkieferkörpers. Dtsch Zahn Mund Kieferheilkd 19:288
136. Upadhyaya P, Dhawan IK, Sidhu S (1965) Replacement of the jaw following excisional surgery for malignant disease of the mandible. Indian J Cancer 2:48
137. Willenegger H, Schenk R (1963) Zum histologischen Bild der sogenannten Primärheilung der Knochenkompakta nach experimentellen Osteotomien am Hund. Experientia 19:593
138. Wilson JSP, Towers JF (1974) Mandibular reconstruction. Proc R Soc Med 67:603
139. Winter L, Lifton JC, McQuillan AS (1945) Embedment of a vitallium mandibular prosthesis as an integral part of the operation for removal of an adamantinoma. Am J Surg 69:318
140. Yoel J (1966) Mandibular reconstruction: methods and results. Int Surg 45:184

Subject Index

Page numbers printed in *italics* refer to an important and detailed description of the concept.

116